Psychological Treatment of
Patients
With Cancer

Clinical Health Psychology Series

Psychological Treatment of Medical Patients in Integrated Primary Care
  Anne C. Dobmeyer

Psychological Treatment of Patients With Cancer
  Ellen A. Dornelas

Psychological Treatment of
Patients
With Cancer

ELLEN A. DORNELAS

CLINICAL HEALTH PSYCHOLOGY SERIES
ELLEN A. DORNELAS, Series Editor

American Psychological Association • Washington, DC

Published by
American Psychological Association
750 First Street, NE
Washington, DC 20002
www.apa.org

To order
APA Order Department
P.O. Box 92984
Washington, DC 20090-2984
Tel: (800) 374-2721; Direct: (202) 336-5510
Fax: (202) 336-5502; TDD/TTY: (202) 336-6123
Online: www.apa.org/pubs/books
E-mail: order@apa.org

In the U.K., Europe, Africa, and the Middle East, copies may be ordered from
American Psychological Association
3 Henrietta Street
Covent Garden, London
WC2E 8LU England

Typeset in Minion by Circle Graphics, Inc., Columbia, MD

Printer: Edwards Brothers Malloy, Lillington, NC
Cover Designer: Mercury Publishing Services, Inc., Rockville, MD

The opinions and statements published are the responsibility of the authors, and such opinions and statements do not necessarily represent the policies of the American Psychological Association.

Library of Congress Cataloging-in-Publication Data

Names: Dornelas, Ellen A., author.
Title: Psychological treatment of patients with cancer / Ellen A. Dornelas.
Other titles: Clinical health psychology series.
Description: First edition. | Washington, DC : American Psychological
   Association, [2018] | Series: Clinical health psychology series | Includes
   bibliographical references and index.
Identifiers: LCCN 2017013399 | ISBN 9781433828058 | ISBN 1433828057
Subjects: | MESH: Neoplasms—psychology | Psychotherapy—methods
Classification: LCC RC271.M4 | NLM QZ 200 | DDC 616.99/40651—dc23 LC record
available at https://lccn.loc.gov/2017013399

British Library Cataloguing-in-Publication Data
A CIP record is available from the British Library.

Printed in the United States of America
First Edition

http://dx.doi.org/10.1037/0000054-000

Contents

CONTENTS

Series Foreword

Mental health practitioners working in medicine represent the vanguard of psychological practice. As scientific discovery and advancement in medicine has rapidly evolved in recent decades, it has been a challenge for clinical health psychology practice to keep pace.

In a fast-changing field, and with a paucity of practice-based research, classroom models of health psychology practice often do not translate well to clinical care. All too often, health psychologists work in silos, with little appreciation of how advancement in one area might inform another. The goal of the Clinical Health Psychology Series is to change these trends and provide a comprehensive yet concise overview of the essential elements of clinical practice in specific areas of health care. The future of 21st-century health psychology depends on the ability of new practitioners to be innovative and to generalize their knowledge across domains. To this end, the series focuses on a variety of topics and provides both a foundation as well as specific clinical examples for mental health professionals who are new to the field.

We have chosen authors who are recognized experts in the field and are rethinking the practice of health psychology to be aligned with modern drivers of health care, such as population health, cost of care, quality of care, and customer experience.

Discussion of the book series began over a cup of coffee in Washington, DC, with Susan Reynolds, senior acquisitions editor at APA Books. I was interested in writing a book about psychological treatment of patients with cancer, and Susan had a vision for a clinical health psychology series written for a practitioner readership. This volume would have never been possible had I not had the great privilege of working with people whose lives have been affected by cancer. To work in psychosocial oncology is also to be humbled in following in the footsteps of many extraordinary leaders who helped this field take shape. It is my hope that this book honors the patients and family members who have helped me to gain great appreciation for the dignity, grace, and resilience of the human spirit in its capacity to cope with cancer.

—Ellen A. Dornelas, PhD
Series Editor

Psychological Treatment of
Patients
With Cancer

Introduction

Although I have been a practicing clinical health psychologist in a hospital setting for many years and have treated quite a few individuals with cancer, I did not become fully immersed in psychosocial oncology until I was hired full-time in a cancer center. As I became immersed in the day-to-day work in this busy urban center, I quickly realized that I needed a brief, easy-to-digest guide that would provide me with information about treating the broad spectrum of patients with cancer.

The challenges of treating the mental health needs of a large volume of high-acuity patients placed great limits on my time. I searched for literature on this topic and found excellent resources, such as the *Quick Reference for Oncology Clinicians: The Psychiatric and Psychological Dimensions of Cancer Symptom Management* (Holland, Greenberg, & Hughes, 2006), published by the American Psychosocial Oncology Society's (APOS) Institute for Research and Education. Indeed, APOS and their international

http://dx.doi.org/10.1037/0000054-001
Psychological Treatment of Patients With Cancer, by E. A. Dornelas
Copyright © 2018 by the American Psychological Association. All rights reserved.

counterpart, the International Psychological Oncology Society, are a welcoming multidisciplinary community devoted to improving the quality of life and the experience of people living with cancer. However, although many excellent books are focused on the psychological experience of people with cancer written for both patients and mental health professionals, I did not find the exact type of book I was searching for. Thus, this volume was written to address what I perceived as a gap in the literature: a book that is succinct but comprehensive in scope such that a mental health professional can build a foundation of knowledge that can generalize to the majority of patients with whom she or he works. This book was written for the practitioner who has a good general understanding of clinical psychology but is new to working with patients who have cancer, or for the practitioner who has worked only with a particular subgroup of oncology patients (e.g., women with breast cancer) and desires to further his or her capability to treat a broader spectrum. My own understanding and clinical work with people who have cancer continues to evolve and has been a tremendously gratifying source of personal and career growth. It is my sincere hope that the information herein will encourage more clinical practitioners to seek additional training in psychosocial oncology. The number of cancer survivors will increase dramatically in the years to come, and it is important that psychology respond by creating the needed workforce.

OVERVIEW OF THIS BOOK

Designed to be practitioner friendly, this book includes a range of psychological interventions aimed at helping patients to cope with the psychological complexity of cancer treatment. The goal of the book is to illustrate the application of psychological approaches in the practice of psychosocial oncology. Although specific approaches are emphasized in each chapter, the reader should try to generalize across topics. Each chapter provides illustrative clinical case examples. Brief descriptions of each chapter follow.

Psychological Treatment for Patients With Cancer follows a structure common to all volumes in the American Psychological Association's Clinical Health Psychology Series. Part I provides a concise overview of cancer and its treatment. Part II focuses on assessment and treatment of common psychological reactions to a cancer diagnosis.

Chapter 1 imparts a basic understanding of cancer and how it progresses. Common categories of cancer, such as breast, prostate, lung, colorectal, brain tumor, sarcoma, lymphoma, leukemia, pancreatic, liver, and certain male and female reproductive cancers, are briefly described. Survival rates for major cancer types are discussed.

Chapter 2 summarizes the main known contributing factors to the development of cancer. The disproportionate impact of cancer on Black/African Americans, Hispanics/Latinos and people who are impoverished in the United States is discussed. Genetic, environmental, and behavioral factors that increase risk for the development and progression of cancer are reviewed, as is the impact of attitudinal and social factors in screening for and coping with cancer.

Chapter 3 provides an overview for nonmedical readers about the major methods used to treat cancer, such as surgery, radiation therapy, and chemotherapy. Commonly used terms in oncology treatment are defined, and some of the psychological aspects of specific cancer treatment are described.

Chapter 4 focuses on depression in patients with cancer. Often, depression goes undetected and untreated. This chapter reviews literature showing that untreated depression may be linked with disease progression. Included in this chapter is a summary of evidence-based psychotherapeutic approaches that have been shown to be effective in treating patients with cancer who are depressed.

Anxiety is the most common psychological symptom encountered in an oncology population. Anxiety and distress fluctuate over the course of treatment, with no strong consensus on the best method or time frame for assessing these constructs. Chapter 5 presents an overview of the continuum of approaches to anxiety treatment for patients with cancer. The Commission on Cancer mandate to screen for distress in patients with cancer is discussed.

Chapter 6 addresses sleep dysregulation and the accompanying fatigue, symptoms that often drive people with cancer to seek psychological treatment. This chapter summarizes the literature in this area and presents an overview of sleep hygiene techniques and specific behavioral strategies to combat fatigue and improve sleep.

Chapter 7 focuses on sexual dysfunction. Cancer and its treatments often affect sexual functioning, but many health care providers are unable to help patients address this concern. The potential influence of side effects of cancer treatments (e.g., mastectomy, hair loss) on body image and intimacy is covered. Strategies for counseling male and female patients with cancer with sexual dysfunction and/or body image disturbance are reviewed.

Chapter 8 discusses the effects the medical condition has on the family of patients with cancer and the role of social support. Spouses and partners of people with cancer often have higher anxiety rates than the patients themselves. The role of the caregiver is taxing, and the resources to address the intense psychological demands of supporting a loved one with a serious health problem are generally inadequate. Most behavioral health clinicians working in psychosocial oncology will counsel patients' family members and therefore need to feel comfortable helping them gain perspective about the diagnosis, assess their resources for support, and develop or maintain a self-care regimen. Caregiving spouses often ask for guidance about how to communicate with their children about a parent who is dying, and this chapter provides some guidelines.

Chapter 9 expounds on the posttreatment psychological sequelae of cancer. There is a growing literature showing that cancer survivorship needs are broader than the psychological aspects and are important to consider from a secondary prevention perspective. The overlap between cancer survivorship and the psychological aftereffects of cancer is also discussed. Fear of reoccurrence, cognitive dysfunction, and the challenges of managing a lifetime of ongoing surveillance are touched on.

Chapter 10 portrays some of the existential themes that abound in oncology care. This chapter reviews the literature on psychological approaches that help people with cancer to accept the inevitability of death and improve quality of life. The controversy surrounding the medical aid in dying movement is explored.

Future directions of practice for cancer care and clinician self-care are discussed in the final chapter, Chapter 11. Many serious psychosocial problems encountered in oncology are neither assessed nor treated, and cancer care needs to be designed to better integrate mental health treatment into the routine delivery of service. Cancer care also requires advanced skill in managing one's own emotions, remaining compassionate, tolerating work overload, and coping with acute distress of patients and their loved ones. Feeling overwhelmed, fatigued, stressed, and/or depressed are all potential signs of compassion fatigue or the loss of enthusiasm for one's life work. This chapter provides cancer clinicians with tools for recognizing burnout and underscores the importance of work–life balance and self-care.

ONE

AN OVERVIEW OF PSYCHOSOCIAL ONCOLOGY

1

An Overview of Cancer for the Mental Health Professional

Cancer is an umbrella term referring to many related diseases. Cancerous tumors are usually solid masses, unless they are blood cancers such as leukemia. Genetics plays an important role in how cancer starts and grows, but this does not mean that all cancers are inherited. Genes control the growth and death of cells. A cell's genes contain DNA, a substance that contains all the cell's operating instructions, including the process for normal cell division. *Mutations* are any abnormal changes in a cell's DNA. Mutations occur because of natural aging, behavioral/ environmental factors (e.g., smoking), familial vulnerability, and other factors. Mutations occur often in cells but are usually repaired by the cell itself or cause the cell to die (a process referred to as *apoptosis*). Cell mutations can be beneficial, harmful, or neutral. Some mutations

http://dx.doi.org/10.1037/0000054-002
Psychological Treatment of Patients With Cancer, by E. A. Dornelas
Copyright © 2018 by the American Psychological Association. All rights reserved.

cause the cell to divide and reproduce in an abnormally fast and uncontrolled way.

Thus, cancer is not a single disease but a category of hundreds of diseases characterized by uncontrolled, abnormal cell division. Cells that are abnormal and divide in an uncontrolled way can *metastasize*, or invade into other areas of the body. Cell mutation may become more aberrant over time. The genetic properties of the original cancer cell evolve, becoming very different from those that develop later or in more distant regions, making cancer more resistant to treatment. For this reason, chemotherapy that works well on the primary tumor may not be as effective in treating metastatic disease. The origin of the type of cell where cancer starts is critical to predicting how the disease will progress. For example, a cancer that has metastasized to the lung but originated in the breast behaves differently from a tumor that originated in the lung. Cancerous cells are greatly heterogeneous. Hematologic (blood) cancers do not form solid tumors. Not all solid tumors are malignant, meaning that they do not metastasize to distant organs. However, brain or central nervous system tumors that grow too large can be deadly if they cannot be removed surgically or contained. The degree to which cancer has progressed is usually assessed by staging.

Clinical staging refers to a physician's interpretation of tests, images, and physical exams. Pathological staging is determined by using this information in addition to surgical results and analysis of characteristics of the tumor itself. Pathologists examine many characteristics of the cell to determine how aggressively the cancer is growing. These features include the level of cell differentiation (how close it appears to the original normal cell), the size of the nucleus, the nucleus-to-cytoplasm (or cellular fluid) ratio, mitotic figures (how many cells are actively dividing), and the architecture of the cell. They also examine the degree to which the cancer has invaded other surrounding tissue, has extended to the basement membrane (meaning the bottom layer of tissue), has created its own blood supply (vascular invasion), and can be found in nearby lymph nodes. The lymph system acts as a filter for the body and is often the first place that a spreading cancer is detected.

CANCER STAGING

Medicine uses a staging system to classify the severity of a majority of cancers (see Table 1.1). Stage 0, I, II, III, and IV are positively correlated with severity of disease.

The tumor, node, and metastasis (TNM) system is one of the most common staging classification systems. *Tumor* incorporates the size of the primary (original) tumor, number of tumors, and grade (degree of abnormality of the tumor cells). *Node* reflects the extent of lymph node involvement. *Metastasis* is determined on the basis of whether the primary tumor has spread outside the original site and whether other secondary tumors exist. Some tumors, such as brain tumors, have no staging system but instead are graded. *Grade* is conceptually similar to stage in that tumors are graded as 1 to 4, with the highest number representing the greatest level of acuity. Cells of low-grade (Grade 1) tumors are well differentiated, whereas high-grade (Grade 4) tumors are undifferentiated and bear little to no resemblance to the original cell.

The most common types of cancer in Americans are breast, prostate, colorectal, and lung cancers. A mental health professional working in hospital-based outpatient oncology will likely see many patients with common cancers. However, psychosocial oncology practices treat a heterogeneous patient population, and it is helpful to have familiarity with many different types of cancer. The mental health professional working with people who have cancer becomes a specialist with some understanding about the broad spectrum of cancers. This is a lifelong learning process because the field is rapidly changing and growing. Brief descriptions of a variety of types of

Table 1.1	
Cancer Staging	
Stage	Definition
0	Carcinoma in situ
I, II, III	The definition of each stage varies depending on the type of cancer, but the higher the stage, the more advanced the cancer.
IV	Advanced cancer that has metastasized to distant tissues or organs.

cancer are given in the following section; however, the list is not exhaustive and is intended as a brief overview upon which to build. Unless otherwise stated, the information in the following section is taken from the American Cancer Society (2013).

BROAD CATEGORIES OF CANCER

Carcinoma refers to the most common category of cancer and is created from epithelial cells that both line and cover organs, as well as the outside of the body. *Sarcomas* are cancers that form in bone and soft tissue. *Osteosarcoma* is the most common type of bone cancer. *Leukemia* is a hematologic or blood cancer caused by the abnormal proliferation of white blood cells (called leukocytes). *Lymphoma* is cancer of the immune system and occurs when another type of blood cell known as lymphocytes abnormally divide and proliferate. *Multiple myeloma* is also a cancer of the immune system that is created through unrestricted growth of plasma cells in bone marrow.

In the sections that follow, examples of common and less common cancers are described. These categories of cancer were chosen to provide information from which the reader can generalize and understand how to access appropriate evidence-based resources for additional information on these or other cancers. Many types of specific cancers are not included due to limitations in the scope of the chapter. Five-year relative survival rates are presented and are calculated as the proportion of people who are alive 5 years after diagnosis, divided by the proportion of the general population of same sex and age who are alive after 5 years. Relative survival rates measured in 5-year increments are useful for epidemiologists to measure progress (or lack thereof) in reducing deaths from cancer over time. Five-year survival rates are not useful in terms of specific predictive value for individuals, but they provide an approximation that should only be taken into consideration in combination with all available clinical information and, ideally, interpreted in context by the patient's physician. Although this statistic is controversial, 5-year survival rates are strongly correlated with mortality rates normalized by incidence, which is generally regarded as a robust, but less commonly used, statistic among nonscientists (Maruvka, Tang, & Michor, 2014).

Breast Cancer

Breast cancer is the most common type of cancer, and more than 232,000 new cases of invasive breast cancer are diagnosed each year in women. Breast cancer occurs rarely in men, with approximately 2,000 new diagnoses made annually in the United States. The numerous categories of breast cancer each have their own course. At the molecular level, breast cancer is many diseases with the common denominator of having originated out of breast tissue. Survival rates differ according to type and stage of cancer. The relative five survival rates for local, regional and advanced breast cancer are 99%, 84%, and 24%, respectively, for an overall 5-year survival rate of 89%, but survival rates should be interpreted with caution because of the variety of factors that influence mortality.

With advances in imaging techniques, more breast cancers are detected at the earliest stages. Ductal carcinoma in situ (DCIS) is Stage 0 preinvasive carcinoma, meaning that abnormal cells are contained within the duct. DCIS has a 30% recurrence rate and a 3% mortality rate. From a mental health professional's perspective, the intensity of anxiety associated with DCIS is not dissimilar to the anxiety of women with advanced cancers. It is important to ascertain both the patients' understanding of their own prognosis as well as the perspective of their treating health care providers. Because women are more likely than men to seek mental health treatment under stress, therapists who treat people with cancer will see many women with invasive breast cancer and many with DCIS.

Invasive ductal carcinoma is the most common type of invasive breast cancer and originates in the milk duct of the breast, then invades into surrounding tissue. Invasive lobular carcinoma is less common and begins in the milk-producing glands or lobules. Invasive lobular carcinoma is less frequently detected on mammogram. Although DCIS and invasive ductal carcinoma produce tumors, other types of breast cancer, for example, inflammatory breast cancer, do not. Inflammatory breast cancer is not common and is characterized by swollen, red, and tender breasts, due to cancerous cells that block lymph vessels. Inflammatory breast cancer is associated with poor prognosis and does not show up on mammogram. Paget's disease refers to cancer of the nipple and is often associated with DCIS. Phyllodes tumors (a rare tumor of the breast's connective tissue) can be benign or malignant. These are likely to recur and can progress to malignancy over time.

Approximately 80% of invasive breast cancers have estrogen and/or progesterone receptors on the tumor. If breast cancer is hormone receptor positive, it is treated with hormones that block estrogen receptors or reduce estrogen levels. In contrast, hormone-receptor-negative breast cancer does not have estrogen and progesterone receptors and does not respond to hormone treatment. About 15% to 20% of invasive breast cancers are characterized by a protein called human epidural growth factor receptor 2, or HER2, in which the cells produce too much HER2 protein. These breast cancers are more aggressive, more often seen in younger women, and respond to drugs that target the HER2 protein, such as Herceptin. Triple positive breast cancer cells are positive for estrogen, progesterone, and an excess of HER2. Triple negative breast cancer cells have no estrogen, progesterone, and no excess HER2. The implication is that HER2 negative breast cancers are more aggressive and difficult to treat because there is no hormonal target to exploit. Although triple negative cancer has a poor prognosis, after 5 years, the survival rates are similar to those of other cancers. The many other types of breast cancer that are not discussed here are less common, and the interested reader is referred to the *American Cancer Society's Breast Cancer Facts & Figures* for more comprehensive review on this topic (American Cancer Society, 2013).

Prostate Cancer

Prostate cancer is the most common type of cancer in men. The prostate is a walnut-shaped gland below the bladder and in front of the rectum. Cancer that starts in a gland is called *adenocarcinoma*, and most prostate cancers are adenocarcinomas. Prostate cancers are most often detected because of a blood test for prostate specific antigen (PSA) or a palpable tumor found by digital rectal exam. Approximately four of five prostate cancers are detected in the local stage, meaning that the cancer has not spread beyond the prostate. Regional stage prostate cancer has spread from the prostate but has not spread to the lymph system or distant areas of the body. Prostate cancer that is biopsied is graded on a scale called a Gleason score, which refers to a method of characterizing the tumor according to how closely the tissue resembles normal prostate tissue. The relative 5-, 10-, and 15-year survival rates for locally or regionally staged prostate cancer are nearly 100%, 99%, and 94%, respectively. Prostate cancers that have not spread have excellent survival rates, but advanced prostate cancer that has metastasized to distant organs, lymph nodes, or bones has a 28% 5-year relative survival rate from time of diagnosis. A therapist treating a patient with prostate cancers should understand the stage of disease. Many men with prostate cancer are understandably anxious because of the diagnosis and/or treatment but have an excellent prognosis. However, common sequelae of treatment include sexual dysfunction (discussed further in Chapter 7, this volume) and incontinence, symptoms that diminish quality of life. Some men diagnosed with advanced prostate cancer feel that their psychological needs are overlooked, with the increasing public recognition that prostate cancer is very treatable. Although it is generally true that people with advanced cancer have different psychological needs from those with less advanced cancer, in the case of prostate cancer, a patient can be negatively impacted if his experience is trivialized or minimized by others unfamiliar with the trajectory of advanced disease. This can also be true of other types of cancer (e.g., thyroid, skin).

Lung Cancer

Lung cancer is the leading cause of cancer-related death in men and women, and about 221,000 new cases of lung cancer are diagnosed each year. Prostate cancer is diagnosed more frequently in men, and breast cancer is diagnosed more frequently in women, making lung cancer the second most common cancer in both men and women. About 6.6% of men and women will be diagnosed with lung or bronchus cancer over their lifetime. Most (> 85%) of lung cancers are non-small cell lung cancers (NSCLC). Non-small cell lung cancers fall into one of three main categories: (a) adenocarcinoma (30%–50%), (b) squamous cell epidermoid carcinoma (20%–25%), or (c) large cell undifferentiated carcinoma (10%–15%). Each category has different treatment implications and prognosis. NSCLC includes other less common types as well. Small cell lung cancer (SCLC) accounts for 10% to 15% of lung cancers and is primarily caused by smoking. The cells found in SCLC tumors multiply rapidly, and in contrast to breast, prostate, and colorectal cancers, lung cancer is difficult to detect in the early stages. The relative 5-year survival rate for lung cancer detected at the earliest stage is nearly 50%, but lung cancer detected at Stage IV is 1%. The U.S. Preventive Services Task Force recommends lung cancer screening for high-risk individuals (i.e., current smokers and former smokers who quit within the past 15 years, ages 55 to 80, with ≥ 30 pack-year smoking history; Moyer & U.S. Preventive Services Task Force, 2014). More than 8 million U.S. citizens meet these screening criteria, and it is estimated that screening can prevent 12,000 lung cancer deaths annually.

Colorectal Cancer

Colorectal cancer is the third leading cause of cancer-related death. More than 90,000 new cases of colon cancer and more than 39,000 new cases of rectal cancer are detected each year. Colorectal cancer refers to cancer of the large intestine or colon; the last several inches of the colon comprise the rectum. The colon is about 5 feet long and thus is the largest part of the digestive system. Most colon cancers begin as benign polyps (noncancerous cells) that have the possibility of becoming cancerous over time. Most (95%), but not all, colon cancers are adenocarcinomas. The proliferation of colonoscopy and fecal immunochemical testing has helped to ensure that more colorectal cancers are found at the earliest and most treatable stages. The incidence of colorectal cancer has dropped by more than 45% since the 1980s (Welch & Robertson, 2016). The overall relative 5-year survival rate for colorectal cancer is 65%.

Pancreatic Cancer

Pancreatic cancer accounts for about 3% of all cancers but has the highest mortality rate of all cancers. The pancreas produces hormones, such as insulin, and enzymes that perform many functions but primarily aid in food digestion. About 95% of pancreatic cancers are adenocarcinomas that originate from exocrine cells. Exocrine pancreatic cancer generally has a poor prognosis, with a 5-year survival rate of less than 15%, even when diagnosed at the earliest stage. People treated with surgical resection of pancreatic tumors have a survival rate of approximately 18 to 20 months. The overall relative 5-year survival rate for exocrine pancreatic cancer at all stages is 6%.

Liver and Bile Duct Cancer

Primary liver and intrahepatic bile duct cancer are not common, compared with other cancers, but the incidence has been increasing over the past 50 years. The liver metabolizes nutrients, contributes to coagulation, secretes bile into the intestine to help absorb fats, and removes toxins from alcohol and drugs from the body. Known risks for liver cancer include hepatitis C virus, hepatitis B virus, cirrhosis, obesity, nonalcoholic fatty liver disease, Type II diabetes, and cigarette smoking. Hepatocellular carcinoma is the most common form of liver cancer. Intrahepatic cholangiocarcinoma or bile duct cancer accounts for about 10% to 20% of primary liver cancers. The 5-year relative survival rate of liver and intrahepatic bile duct cancer at all stages is 17%.

Ovarian Cancer

Ovarian cancer accounts for about 3% of cancers among women but causes more deaths than any other cancer of the female reproductive system. More than 20,000 American women are diagnosed with ovarian cancer each year. More than 85% of ovarian cancers are epithelial. Other types of ovarian cancers develop in the lining of the fallopian tube and primary peritoneal cavity (develops from cells in the lining of the pelvis and abdomen). Other less common types of ovarian cancer also exist. Eight of 10 ovarian cancers are diagnosed at advanced stages. The 20% of women with early-stage ovarian cancer have relative 5-year survival rates of greater than 90%, but the overall survival rate is 45% because the disease is usually diagnosed after it has metastasized. Cancer antigen 125 (CA 125) is a protein found on the surface of ovarian cancer cells and in blood and is used as a tumor marker to indicate response to treatment or recurrence. Rising CA 125 levels can indicate progression of disease, but this is an imperfect marker and should be interpreted with caution in the context of multiple other factors. Ovarian cancer metastasizes in the peritoneal cavity, and treatments for advanced disease often target the uterus, bowel, or surrounding areas.

Skin Cancer

Skin cancer is the most common type of cancer. Basal cell carcinoma is the most common form of skin cancer; squamous cell carcinoma is the second most common. Although melanoma accounts for just 2% of skin cancers, it is the most serious and is the primary cause of death from skin cancer. The cells that produce melanin, which gives pigment to skin, are prone to mutation when exposed to ultraviolet radiation from sun exposure or tanning beds. Although most skin cancers occur later in life, increasing numbers of young people are developing the disease. The overall relative 5-year survival rate for skin melanoma is 92%, but for Stage IV disease drops to about 15% to 20%.

Leukemia

Leukemia is a systemic disease and refers to a cancer of the early forming blood cells, usually the white blood cells. Blood is primarily made up of plasma, red blood cells, white blood cells, and platelets. Blood brings oxygen to the organs, fights infection, regulates body temperature, filters waste products via the kidney and liver, and forms clots to prevent blood loss. White blood cells are leukocytes and prevent infection. The majority of white blood cells are neutrophils, sometimes called the "immediate response" of the body. Lymphocytes are the other type of white blood cells and are the foundation of the immune response. As a general rule, leukemia is either acute or chronic and either granulocyte or lymphocyte. Acute leukemia that is untreated progresses very rapidly in months, whereas chronic leukemia is much slower to progress. The relative 5-year survival rate for all subtypes of leukemia combined is approximately 62%, but there is wide variation between subtypes.

Lymphoma

Lymphoma is the most common presentation of hematologic malignancy. Lymphoma occurs when lymphocyte cells mutate and proliferate in both blood and the lymph system. Lymphoma can also originate from other types of cells but is most often associated with lymphocyte malignancy. The two broad categories of lymphoma are Hodgkin lymphoma (HL) and non-Hodgkin lymphoma (NHL). Many types of lymphoma exist within these categories. The majority (90%) of cases of lymphoma are NHL. The relative 5-year survival rate for HL is 88%; for NHL, it is approximately 72%. Approximately 8,500 new cases of HL and 72,000 new cases of NHL are diagnosed each year in the United States. The many categories of NHL and prognosis vary widely, depending on the type and stage of disease. The overall relative 5-year survival rate for HL is 86%. Hodgkin disease or HL is named after Dr. Thomas Hodgkin, who identified the disease.

Multiple Myeloma

Multiple myeloma occurs because plasma cells (mainly found in bone marrow) mutate and proliferate. Many organs can be affected by multiple myeloma, but bone lesions are most common. Bone pain is the most common symptom of multiple myeloma, but the disease is also associated with kidney failure, anemia, and neurologic problems, as well as susceptibility to pneumonia and other infections. Approximately 24,000 new diagnoses of multiple myeloma are made each year. Multiple myeloma is the second most prevalent hematologic cancer following NHL. The overall relative 5-year survival rate is 45% but varies depending on the stage of diagnoses and presentation of disease.

Osteosarcoma and Sarcoma

Most cancers such as breast, lung, and colorectal originate from epithelial cells and are referred to as *carcinoma*. By contrast, *sarcoma* is cancer that originates from other tissues (e.g., bone, cartilage, fat). Osteosarcoma is cancer of the bone and occurs most often in the femur and tibia, usually in young adults or children. The overall relative 5-year survival rate for localized osteosarcoma is better than 90% but drops to 30% disease diagnosed in later stages. Survival rates vary widely depending on stage of disease and characteristics of the tumor. Soft tissue sarcoma occurs in connective tissue. Approximately 9,500 new diagnoses of soft tissue sarcoma occur each year in the United States. The overall relative 5-year survival rate is highly variable depending on the origin and characteristics of the tumor and stage of disease. People diagnosed with AIDS are at risk for Kaposi's sarcoma, which occurs in the blood vessels of the skin and mucus tissue.

Bladder and Kidney Cancer

Urologic cancers occur most often in the bladder, and approximately 76,000 Americans are diagnosed with bladder cancer each year. Bladder cancer is diagnosed in more than 58,000 men and 18,000 women each year. Older age is a primary risk factor for bladder cancer, and 90% of cases are diagnosed in adults over the age of 55 years. The overall relative 5-year survival rate for all stages of bladder cancer is 77%. About 62,000 people in the United States, most often men and older adults, are diagnosed with kidney cancer. The most common type of kidney cancer is renal cell carcinoma. Early stage localized kidney cancer has very good 5-year relative rates of 81% or better, whereas kidney cancer diagnosed at the most advanced stage has a 5-year survival rate of 8%.

Brain Tumors

Tumors that originate in the brain do not usually spread to distant organs but are destructive as they grow. Tumors that start in glial cells include glioblastoma, astrocytoma, ependymoma, and oligodendroglioma. Brain tumors are graded, rather than staged, by the level of differentiation of the cell and the rate at which it grows. Meningiomas account for approximately one of three brain tumors and originate in the tissue surrounding the brain or spinal cord. The multiple other types of primary brain tumors and pituitary tumors have great variety in histology (i.e., the structure of the cancer cell examined under the microscope). Brain tumors and their treatment can cause a great deal of cognitive impairment and physical dysfunction, or they may be relatively asymptomatic. Neuropsychologists are often involved in assessing cognitive functioning for patients with brain tumors. Common symptoms found in people treated for brain tumor (e.g., headaches, seizures, hearing or vision loss, fatigue, memory deficits) have a significant psychological adjustment component. Both patients and caregivers of people who have brain tumors can benefit from psychological support.

HOW MUCH ONCOLOGY EDUCATION DOES THE MENTAL HEALTH PROFESSIONAL NEED?

Compared with many other areas of clinical health psychology, the field of oncology is more complex and potentially involves any system of the body. Most mental health professionals wish there were an easy way to gain the necessary understanding of the field. Therapists working in oncology will encounter many presentations of cancer that are unfamiliar, which will provide a window into the patient's perspective on the struggle and challenges of understanding their diagnosis. A simple educational strategy is to ask patients directly about their understanding of their cancer and supplement this information with a follow-up call to the medical or radiation oncologist. Physicians and other providers are typically grateful to have a mental health professional participate in patient care and will usually give brief education about the patient's cancer if directly asked. It is also helpful to use credible sources, such as the American Cancer Society or National Cancer Institute websites, for additional information about the specifics of any given cancer.

2

Etiology and Sociocultural Factors Related to Cancer

Trends in cancer care show that the *incidence* (number of new cases in a given time period) of cancer will increase by 45% by 2030 and that the number of cancer survivors (also called *prevalence*) will increase by 30% by 2032. In 2016, there were 13.7 million total cancer survivors, but this number is projected to increase to 18 million by 2022. Cancer incidence has increased primarily because of gains in life expectancy over the past century. A baby born in 1900 in the United States had a lifespan of 47 years, but children born today will live to about 78 years. In the United States, the population over the age of 65 is expected to nearly double from 48 million to 88 million by 2050 (He, Goodkind, & Kowal, 2016). The dramatic increase in life expectancy is due primarily to victories in the war on infectious diseases, such as pneumonia, flu, and tuberculosis through advances in medicine and public health. Americans today live much longer and are

http://dx.doi.org/10.1037/0000054-003
Psychological Treatment of Patients With Cancer, by E. A. Dornelas

susceptible to the development of health conditions such as cardiovascular disease and cancer that, in turn, are tied to aging and health behaviors.

CAUSES OF CANCER

In addition to aging, cancer can have many different etiologies that include genetic vulnerability, health behaviors (e.g., tobacco use, alcohol use, poor diet, sedentary behavior), and infection. Environmental exposures to radiation, benzene, asbestos, Agent Orange, and other agents (known as *carcinogens*) also increase risk for cancer.

Genetics

All cancer is genetic in origin because cancer represents genetic change in a cell. The germ line genome is encoded in germ cells (eggs and sperm) and determines traits that will be inherited, such as height and hair color. Only 10% to 15% of cancers are hereditary germ line mutations. Somatic cells are not transmitted from parent to child. Somatic mutations are acquired and are the drivers of the single rogue cell that mutates and proliferates. Whole genome sequencing for cancer has undergone an evolution since the publication of the Human Genome Project (International Human Genome Sequencing Consortium, 2004), and with each passing year, an increasing number of somatic mutations are linked to specific tumor types. The clinical applications of whole genome sequencing are only in the earliest stages of development, but this technology makes it possible to identify somatic markers of the tumor and develop drugs that target the specific marker. The difference between the toxic chemotherapies of 30 years ago, compared with today's targeted therapies for somatic mutation, has been likened to the difference in effect between a grenade and a sniper. Personalized cancer therapy based on genomic sequencing targets the mutant cell but not healthy tissue. But genomic sequencing is still a nascent science, and far more is unknown in this field than has been discovered. Many somatic mutations exist for which no targeted therapy has been developed. Patients who undergo germ line testing receive genetics counseling from a professionally trained genetics counselor who explains risk for disease if germ line mutations exist. Results of genome sequencing in clinical medicine are typically explained by the physician who ordered the test; if a somatic mutation is discovered but no drug or clinical trial is available, the patient may derive no direct benefit from molecular testing.

Infection

Infectious causes of cancer refer to viruses, such as the human papilloma virus (HPV). HPV is a broad category of more than 150 viruses that are spread by contact. Most often, the immune system attacks HPV viruses, and the majority of people who have a form of HPV never develop cancer. However, some types of HPV are linked to cervical cancers, as well as to head and mouth cancers. HPV vaccines were approved in 2006 and can be used to vaccinate young girls and boys. Epstein–Barr virus (EBV) causes mononucleosis, and once infected, people carry the virus for the rest of their life. Most people remain asymptomatic, but in some cases, EBV is related to cancer that develops at the back of the nose and certain types of lymphoma. Hepatitis B and C (HBV and HCV, respectively) are viral infections that can damage the liver and cause liver cancer. Early detection of HBV and HCV can allow for preventive steps to reduce risk for liver damage and cancer. Human immunodeficiency virus (HIV) and human herpes virus-8 (HHV-8) can cause Kaposi sarcoma and some types of lymphoma. Other viral infections are also associated with cancer but are less common and not well understood.

Bacteria and parasites can also cause infections associated with cancer. *Helicobacter pylori* (H. pylori) is a bacterium commonly found in the stomach and is typically asymptomatic, but in some people, it can cause stomach cancer. This is rare in the United States but more common globally. *Chlamydia trachomatis* is also a common bacterium of the female reproductive system that is usually not harmful but is associated with higher risk of cervical cancer. Certain parasites can also cause cancer, but this generally occurs in other parts of the world. Americans are generally only at risk for this if they travel abroad in certain regions. Several key modifiable causes of cancer are described in the following section.

Tobacco

Tobacco use remains the leading preventable cause of cancer. Cigarettes contain more than 70 known carcinogens and are responsible for 80% to 90% of lung cancers. It is intuitive that tobacco would be associated with risk for all cancers of the respiratory system. Less well recognized is that tobacco use is also associated with increased risk for most types of cancers, especially those found in the head, neck, breast, and gastrointestinal system. Screening for tobacco use and appropriate treatment and referral is part of recommended standard care in oncology. Although many people develop cancer long after they stop smoking, a substantial number continue to smoke after a cancer diagnosis. It is difficult for a patient to admit to ongoing tobacco use after a cancer diagnosis. Paradoxically, the stress of a cancer diagnosis makes it all the more difficult to stop smoking. Individual counseling for smoking cessation is effective (Lancaster & Stead, 2017) and appropriate for oncology patients.

Alcohol

Alcohol is related to increased risk for esophageal and other cancers of the gastrointestinal system. There is a dose–response relationship between alcohol consumption and some types of cancer. Alcohol contains many carcinogens, including acetaldehyde. Alcohol is most dangerous to the parts of the body it contacts directly (e.g., the oral cavity, esophagus, colon, rectum, and liver). Alcohol has also been linked to breast cancer. Women who have two to five drinks daily have 1.5 times the risk of developing breast cancer compared with those who abstain from alcohol (Kotsopoulos et al., 2010). This finding is complicated in light of studies showing a cardio-protective effect from light to moderate alcohol consumption. The threshold for increased cancer risk from alcohol use occurs when consumption is greater than approximately 1 drink/day for women and 1.5 drinks/day for men. It is challenging to find strong epidemiological data on current alcohol abuse in newly diagnosed patients with cancer, but histories of lifetime alcohol abuse are noteworthy and suggest the need to incorporate screening into routine delivery of care (Mehnert et al., 2014). The CAGE questionnaire (Ewing, 1984) is a valid method of assessing alcohol use in an oncology population. The questions are, Have you ever felt you needed to Cut down on your alcohol use? Have people Annoyed you by criticizing you about drinking? Have you ever felt Guilty about drinking? Have you Ever felt you needed to have a drink first thing in the morning? Few studies focus on concurrent alcohol treatment for oncology patients, but heavy drinking complicates cancer treatment. Mental health professionals working in psychosocial oncology have a unique window of opportunity to address problem drinking and alcohol dependence at a point when the patient may be highly motivated to make a lifestyle change.

Diet

The American diet entails risk for cancer because it is often filled with carbohydrates, saturated fats, and trans fats and is low in fiber and fruits and vegetables. Processed, preserved, and cured meats are associated with cancer. A plethora of studies have focused on dietary factors and cancer. For example, researchers have studied the effects of tea, genetically modified food, vegetarian and vegan diet, artificial sweeteners, dietary supplements, soy, irradiated foods, fish, coffee, and antioxidants. However, the evidence is often conflicting and confusing. Anyone with a new cancer diagnosis (especially people are prone to anxiety) can become distraught and overwhelmed by the contradictory evidence related to diet and cancer. In general, most oncologists would agree that keeping body mass index (BMI) to a normal range and eating a Mediterranean diet and omega-3 fatty acids reduce risk for chronic diseases, including many types of cancers (Kushi et al., 2012). Dieticians certified to treat oncology patients play a key role in preventing malnutrition, intervene to prevent wasting, and help patients who require feeding tubes. A percutaneous endoscopic gastrostomy feeding tube is used to prevent malnutrition for people with cancers, such as those found in the head and neck. Weaning from a feeding tube can be challenging, and people fear choking due to difficulty swallowing. Mental health professionals working in tandem with oncology dieticians can deploy principles of exposure and desensitization to address this common problem.

Sedentary Lifestyle

Obesity contributes to about 15% to 20% of all cancer-related mortality (Kushi et al., 2012). The 2012 American Cancer Society guidelines recommend a physically active lifestyle. The American Cancer Society recommends that adults engage in at least 150 minutes of moderate intensity or 75 minutes of high-intensity exercise a week. Patients who were sedentary before being diagnosed with cancer are advised to increase their level of physical activity once treatment is completed. Yet, this is difficult for most Americans.

Unlike cardiac rehabilitation, cancer care does not typically include a similar type of posttreatment rehabilitation exercise program. The functional capabilities of people with cancer vary widely. Many people cope with general or specific impairments and could benefit from impairment-driven cancer rehabilitation (Silver, Baima, & Mayer, 2013).

Physical activity as a form of secondary risk prevention has a different focus and target population than does impairment-driven cancer rehabilitation. LIVESTRONG at the YMCA was developed by the LIVESTRONG Foundation and is a 12-week physical activity program for people diagnosed with cancer. This type of program is effective in terms of providing instruction and motivation to begin an exercise regimen, as well as providing a support function by connecting cancer survivors with each other. Evidence also suggests that continuing a physician-approved exercise regimen during cancer treatment helps to improve mood and quality of life and may even improve response to chemotherapy (Friedenreich, Neilson, Farris, & Courneya, 2016).

Sun and Ultraviolet Light

Sun exposure and use of tanning beds are health risk behaviors that increase risk of skin cancer. Strong evidence indicates that ultraviolet light (UVR) is the primary risk factor for skin cancer. Use of a tanning bed before the age of 35 increases risk for melanoma by 75%. Skin cancer is the most common form of cancer, and the number of new cases of melanoma is increasing by approximately 3% annually in the United States (Tripp, Watson,

Balk, Swetter, & Gershenwald, 2016). One out of three high school seniors and more than half of college students report having used a tanning bed (Guy et al., 2014). Dangerous UVR exposure is more prevalent in women (particularly White women) than in men, and evidence indicates that tanning can be addictive (Mosher & Danoff-Burg, 2010). Education alone is not sufficient to prevent persistent tanning in cancer survivors. Tanned skin has been associated with health, youth, and beauty in U.S. culture for many decades. Multicomponent psychological intervention that incorporates appearance-based messages, photo-aging information, and promotion of alternative behaviors (e.g., use of sunless tanner) can influence outcomes related to perceived susceptibility to skin cancer, attitudes about tanning, use of protective clothing, skin self-exam, and reduction in exposure to UVR. The clinical applicability of this research to cancer survivors needs to be determined (Wu et al., 2016). Cultural norms about health risk behaviors and preventive screening influence susceptibility to many types of cancer, a topic discussed in the section that follows.

Sociocultural Factors Related to Cancer

Cultural values play a critical role in how cancer is conceptualized and the stage at which it is detected. Some cultural subgroups view certain cancers as shameful or stigmatic for the family in some subcultures. For example, some families who have a high degree of genetic vulnerability to cancer consider their family to be cursed (Baider & Surbone, 2010). Many myths about cancer persist. Within some cultural subgroups, cancer is perceived to be contagious, such that a husband could refuse to sleep with his wife after a cancer diagnosis. It is challenging to determine the relative contribution of poverty, low educational levels, and lack of health care access to cancer disparities. Education has a strong and consistent relationship to cancer morbidity and mortality. Low education levels are associated with poor nutrition, sedentary lifestyle, obesity, tobacco, and alcohol abuse. Poverty has both direct and indirect effects on health. For example, the working poor are less likely to have paid sick leave or to be able to take time off for preventive health screens. Baider and Surbone (2010) made the point that education is prevention, and many efforts in eliminating health disparities focus on education and advocacy for cancer prevention in underrepresented and marginalized groups.

Compared with other racial groups, Black men and women are at increased risk for many cancers and have the highest death rates from cancer. Black Americans are also less likely to enroll in clinical research trials. The reasons for racial disparities in cancer risk and outcomes are complex, multidirectional, multifactorial, and not completely understood. Early developmental factors, such as diet and physical activity, contribute to obesity, which disproportionately affects Blacks. Black Americans are more likely to be impoverished and more have a low educational level; when these factors are controlled, the degree of difference between Blacks and Whites is reduced. However, there are also differences in the types of cancers that affect racial subgroups; for instance, Black women are more likely to be diagnosed with triple negative breast cancer, a more aggressive and difficult-to-treat disease. More research on the prevention and treatment of cancer in underrepresented racial minorities is needed.

Latinos who move to the United States increase their risk of cancer by nearly 40%. Latinos are the fastest growing demographic group in the United States. This heterogeneous group is widely diverse and includes Mexicans, Puerto Ricans, Cubans, Brazilians, and a multitude of immigrant groups from Central and South America. Latino subgroups are greatly diverse in race and ethnicity, so it is difficult to generalize. But in general, Hispanic Americans are at greater risk for some gynecological cancers, as well as liver cancer. Hispanics are less likely to have preventive vaccinations, such as HPV and hepatitis, and this in turn contributes to greater risk for head/neck and liver cancer, respectively.

The impact of attitudinal and social factors in screening for and coping with cancer is significant. Many cancers are detected late because of reluctance to undergo screening tests, such as colonoscopy, pap smears, or mammograms. Community outreach efforts via mobile mammography, community health fairs, and targeted campaigns aimed at places of worship have been successful in the United States at increasing access to health services and knowledge about the importance of preventive health screening.

Perception of some cancers is adversely affected by attitudes. People with lung cancer often face stigma and feel judged, regardless of whether they smoked cigarettes. Attitudes greatly affect whether people will see a doctor regularly, undergo recommended health screenings, and seek appropriate medical help when symptoms occur. Four attitudinal factors related to seeking medical help are fatalism, trust, procrastination/avoidance, and intention (Fischer, Dornelas, & DiLorenzo, 2013). People who are fatalistic and agree that "when your time is up, that's it, there's nothing you can do" tend to be less likely to engage in necessary health screening tests (M. Cohen, 2013). The Tuskegee experiment[1] is most often cited as a reason that African Americans may be more likely to distrust the health care system. However, this reticence varies by region, generation, level of health care access, and other factors. A mailed survey of Connecticut residents showed that Black respondents were more likely than Whites to endorse trust for their doctor (Dornelas, Fischer, & DiLorenzo, 2014). The tendency to procrastinate or avoid medical appointments may be an important reason that many preventable cancers are detected at advanced stages. Finally, intention is a strong predictor of health behaviors. Psychological interventions that influence intention have great potential for primary and secondary cancer prevention. Many of the risk factors for cancer can be controlled. Avoiding tobacco use, alcohol abuse, maintaining a healthy BMI, and moderate, regular exercise each week would prevent up 70% of new cancer cases in the United States, according to a study of a cohort of White Americans (Song & Giovannucci, 2016).

---

[1] The Tuskegee experiment was conducted by the U.S. government and studied the progression of untreated syphilis in African American men in Alabama. The study lasted 4 decades, but participants were never treated with penicillin, even though it became the standard of care in the late 1940s. This biomedical research study was widely condemned when it became public in the 1970s and led to more robust protection of human subjects through federal law.

3

Standard Medical Treatments for Cancer and Patient Decision Making

This chapter provides an overview for nonmedical readers about cancer treatment modalities, including surgery, radiation therapy, and chemotherapy. Terms such as *adjuvant, neoadjuvant,* or *palliative* are not necessarily familiar to behavioral health specialists who are new to working in oncology. *Adjuvant therapies* are used in combination with the primary treatment to maximize effectiveness and keep cancer from recurring or progressing. *Neoadjuvant therapy* is administered before the primary treatment, often with the goal of minimizing the extent of surgery and sometimes to demonstrate the degree to which the tumor will respond to chemotherapy prior to surgical removal. The goal of *palliative care* is to improve quality of life rather than to cure cancer. Palliative care is discussed in more detail in Chapter 10. The goal of this chapter is to provide an overview of cancer treatment and potential psychological pitfalls that arise with specific treatments. Technological advances and cultural change

http://dx.doi.org/10.1037/0000054-004
Psychological Treatment of Patients With Cancer, by E. A. Dornelas

over the past decade have led to more people making decisions about their cancer care. The burgeoning literature about health care decision making suggests that clinicians working in oncology benefit from having a framework about how to counsel and support people who need to make complex health-related choices.

SURGERY

Surgery refers to the removal of an abnormal lesion or tumor and remains the primary method by which solid tumors are excised. Clean margins mean that an additional rim surrounding the tumor is removed with no evidence of cancerous cells. Surgery is the treatment of choice for many cancers, such as non–small cell lung cancer. Often, surgery is the primary treatment for people with early-stage cancers. Among women with early-stage breast cancer, approximately 35.5% are treated with mastectomy and 64.5% are treated with breast-conserving surgery (Kummerow, Du, Penson, Shyr, & Hooks, 2015). The numbers of prophylactic mastectomies, oophorectomies, and other preventive surgeries have increased dramatically as more deleterious genetic mutations are identified. About 54.5% of men diagnosed with low-risk prostate cancer opt for surgery rather than active surveillance (Gray, Lin, Jemal, & Efstathiou, 2014). Within the last 30 days of life, more than one out of four patients undergo invasive procedures for incurable cancers (Chen et al., 2016). Length of time and ability to recover from surgery involves many factors, including type and extent of surgery, removal of lymph nodes, other preexisting conditions, and complications. Some surgeries, such as mastectomy, can involve reconstructive surgery, which in turn may take place through additional surgeries or procedures (e.g., placement of tissue expanders) taking place over the course of up to a year. Some types of cancer involve only surgery, and from the patient's perspective, the surgeon may be the primary doctor that they associate with their cancer care.

Psychologically, immediate and long-term response to surgery involves many factors, including preexisting psychological functioning, pain control, the degree to which the patient experiences functional impairment (e.g., needing a colostomy, being restricted from driving), and support from friends and family. Mental health professionals can be consulted when patients are struggling with medical decision making related to surgery (described in more detail later in this chapter) or adjustment to the surgery itself. Psychological reactions to major surgeries, such as mastectomy, vary widely. It is typical to mourn the loss of the integrity of the body, question health care decisions after the fact, or feel otherwise greatly psychologically impacted by surgery. Although some people are greatly affected, others find that the psychological of aspect surgery diminishes in intensity over time or has little effect on their mental health at all.

CHEMOTHERAPY

Chemotherapy evokes many connotations but simply means drug or medication therapy. Chemotherapy is used for many purposes, including to kill off cancerous cells, to keep cancer from spreading, or to slow it down and/or to provide symptom relief. Chemotherapy is usually delivered by intravenous (IV) infusion over a period of time as short as 30 minutes or as long as 14 hours. Continuous infusions from an IV pump can last for up to a week. Often, people undergoing chemotherapy have central venous catheters surgically implanted into the chest or other parts of the body to facilitate the delivery of the infusion. A port is one type of central venous catheter. Side effects of chemotherapy vary widely depending on the types and amount of drug utilized. Patients often have an image of a patient undergoing chemotherapy as a person who has lost their hair, suffers nausea, weight loss, and fatigue, and indeed, these are common side effects. However, depending on multiple factors, many people experience minimal side effects and report that chemotherapy is less taxing than they anticipated. As patients undergo additional chemotherapy treatments, the level of toxicity increases and more side effects may be experienced as treatment progresses.

Many other methods of chemotherapy delivery exist, in addition to IV infusion. *Oral chemotherapy* refers to pills or liquids that are typically self-administered at home. *Intrathecal chemotherapy* is delivered to the cerebrospinal fluid via the spine or a port placed under the skin on the head during surgery. Chemotherapy can be injected into the muscle, given regionally into a specific area or organ, or injected into the lesion itself. Chemotherapy can be delivered topically on the skin. Medical oncologists oversee the delivery of chemotherapy and long-term delivery and coordination of oncological care.

IMMUNOTHERAPY

Immunotherapy is viewed by many oncologists as the future of cancer care. It is a form of drug therapy that boosts the body's immune response in a general or cancer-specific way to slow or stop the spread of some types of cancer. The primary types of immunotherapy are monoclonal antibodies, immune checkpoint inhibitors, cancer vaccines, oncolytic viruses, and other nonspecific immunotherapies. Monoclonal antibodies are manufactured antibodies that target antigens (a type of protein) specific to the cancer cell; they are increasingly used to treat some types of breast cancer, leukemia, lymphoma, and other types of cancer. Immune checkpoint inhibitors activate or inactivate molecules on certain immune cells (checkpoints), which help to identify cells as self or other (foreign to the body). As an example, immunotherapy can target checkpoint proteins such as PD-1 and PD-L1 to stimulate the body's own immune system to destroy cancerous cells. Some types of melanoma and small cell lung cancer are treated with immune checkpoint inhibitors. Cancer vaccines can prevent some cancers (e.g., vaccine for the human papilloma virus) or treat cancer. Oncolytic virotherapy uses genetically engineered viruses to destroy cancer cells directly and stimulate the immune system to fight the cancer. Virotherapy can cause cell lysis (destruction of the cancerous cell) or apoptosis (initiation of cell self-destruction sequence). A virus within a cancerous cell takes advantage of the malignant cell's ability to proliferate and multiply, and replicates to destroy cancerous cells without destroying healthy tissue. Some types of viral therapy destroy the cell's vasculature system and/or stimulate production of cytokines, molecules that stimulate the immune system to produce natural killer cells to destroy malignant tumor tissue. Immunotherapy shows great promise as a treatment with fewer side effects than traditional chemotherapy and can be used in combination with other treatments to use the immune system to function more effectively to destroy cancerous cells.

CHEMO-BRAIN

Many factors affect the influence of chemotherapy on mental health functioning, including premorbid psychological functioning, experience of side effects (e.g., fatigue, nausea), level of social support, and type and stage of disease. Some types of chemotherapy (e.g., hormonal therapy, steroids, interferon) are associated with increased risk for anxiety and depression. Many people undergoing adjuvant chemotherapy also have complaints of cognitive loss, especially involving short-term memory and executive function. This has been termed *chemotherapy-associated cognitive impairment*, or colloquially, "chemo-brain," and can significantly impair everyday function. Many people receiving chemotherapy have subjective complaints of cognitive loss, depending on many factors, including the type of cancer, stage, and treatment. Some chemotherapeutic agents cross the blood–brain barrier, and in some cases an argument can be made for a direct effect of chemotherapy on executive functioning. Other variables, such as preexisting cognitive functioning, older age, genetic vulnerability, coexisting depression, and fatigue, also are implicated as contributors. The effect of chemotherapy on cognitive functioning has been difficult to study. In-depth assessment of baseline cognitive functioning before treatment is not typically feasible because patients are understandably anxious to get started on lifesaving chemotherapy. Therefore, careful study of the potential impact of cancer treatment on the brain is needed. Although key preliminary studies have been conducted, as yet, evidence-based interventions for chemotherapy-associated cognitive impairment have not been conducted (Ganz, 2016).

RADIATION THERAPY

Radiation is a form of energy. The average person is exposed to radiation every day via sunlight, when using a microwave or watching television, or when undergoing x-ray imaging. *Ionizing radiation* refers to high-energy electromagnetic waves that cause electrons to become detached from atoms and molecules, thus changing their structure. Radiation oncology therapy injures the DNA of cancer cells, which in turn reduces cellular proliferation and/or triggers cell death thereby shrinking a tumor. Radiation therapy can be delivered by an external beam using a machine, internally by placing radioactive material inside the body (brachytherapy), or systemically by ingesting radioactive material, such as radioactive iodine, or injecting material intravenously that travels to cancerous cells. External beam radiation is usually delivered via a linear accelerator.

Radiation oncologists are physicians who deliver radiation therapy treatment. They are assisted by radiation physicists, who have master's or doctoral-level training, maintain the machines that deliver radiation treatment, and work with radiation oncologists to develop treatment plans. Medical dosimetrists are a key part of the radiation oncology team who calculate the dose of radiation therapy needed to treat the tumor. Radiation therapists administer radiation therapy; patients come to know these staff well because treatment is usually delivered over a period of weeks. A simulation of the radiation therapy treatment plan is conducted before beginning treatment to ensure that the treatment is reproducible and to create any needed immobilization devices or molds. Plastic molds are used for patients with head and neck tumors to ensure that the patient does not move at all.

Psychological effects of radiation therapy may be nonexistent or profound. People who undergo treatment that requires them to be immobilized in a way that can feel claustrophobic, confining, or invasive can find the experience very stressful. Radiation treatment typically occurs over a period of weeks, and most people desensitize after repeated exposure. But for those already predisposed to anxiety, radiation treatment can precipitate panic attacks and acute anxiety.

BONE MARROW TRANSPLANT

Some people with leukemia and lymphoma cancers are candidates for bone marrow transplant. This method implants healthy bone marrow stem cells from the patient's own body or a donor. Total body radiation to suppress the immune system is used before the procedure. Autologous transplant requires the patient's own bone marrow or stem cells. Allogenic transplant utilizes donor cells. Bone marrow transplant is intensive treatment. The length of stay in the hospital and recovery time vary widely from person to person, depending on the type of procedure and potential complications following transplant.

THE GENOMIC ERA OF ONCOLOGY TREATMENT

Cancer, by definition, refers to genetic mutation and the proliferation of previously normal cells. Increasingly, the genetic composition of cancerous cells is analyzed immediately to determine whether genetic markers can identify how the cancer is likely to progress, whether it will respond to standard therapy, and if it is appropriate for specific targeted therapies. Whole genome testing is a technology to analyze the entire DNA sequence. Tumor sequencing tests allow molecular pathologists to determine whether a gene has been changed or deleted, or whether additional copies of it have been made. *Precision medicine* refers to the aim of personalizing medical treatment such that is tailored to the individual's unique genetic characteristics. This information can guide treatment decisions and provide information to match the patient to the right treatment and/or clinical trial. Most mental health professionals working in psychosocial oncology, as well as most patients, do not have the foundation of knowledge needed to understand basic concepts in genomics and thus may not fully appreciate the potential ethical, legal, and psychological implications of whole genome sequencing. Fowler (2016) argued for the need for "genomic literacy" and created http://genomicsforeveryone.org as a course designed to educate the public toward more informed personal decision making and public health policies.

DECISION MAKING

People with a new diagnosis of cancer are called upon to make many important decisions in an era when a high volume of information is available via the Internet but is not necessarily easily understood. Men with slow-growing prostate cancer choose between active treatment via surgery and/or radiation therapy versus surveillance. Women with breast cancer make decisions about whether to undergo lumpectomy, bilateral mastectomy, unilateral mastectomy, and reconstructive surgery. Patients with metastatic disease and/or their caregivers reach a point where they need to decide to continue active treatment or transition to palliative care only. Often patients have rote memorization of the survival rates for their particular cancer as explained to them by their physician, but many factors influence their understanding of the relevance of this information to their personal situation. Cancer has its own language, and it is challenging to understand the language and terms that describe the disease and its potential treatments. The majority of people lack the quantitative ability to fully understand personal risk (Reyna, Nelson, Han, & Dieckmann, 2009). Even among people who have excellent quantitative skills, the fear associated with cancer can impede the ability to process medical information quickly and logically. Furthermore, complex medical decisions are influenced by emotions and perceptions of personal risk as well as understanding of the potential benefits and risks. Fuzzy trace theorizes that patients need to understand the gist of all the information to make an informed decision (Reyna, Nelson, Han, & Pignone, 2015). The essential task of the cancer survivor is to obtain the gist at every important decision-making stage.

DECISIONS ABOUT PARTICIPATION IN CANCER CLINICAL RESEARCH TRIALS

The average mental health professional has limited or basic knowledge about therapeutic cancer clinical trials. *Phase I* clinical trials are those in which a new treatment is used for the first time in humans; they have no control group. Patients with cancer who have exhausted their treatment options may become eligible for Phase I clinical trials. The objective of the Phase I study is to understand the best dose for humans. Phase I studies are typically short term. The potential therapeutic benefit for an individual patient is unknown, and these trials offer a last hope with no assurance of benefit and generally higher levels of potential risk compared with later stage trials. Phase I trials are key to the advancement of knowledge about how to treat the disease. *Phase II* trials examine a treatment's efficacy and may have a control group. Oncology trials typically compare an experimental treatment versus the best-known standard treatment for the condition. Participation in Phase II trials can last for years, and the likelihood of benefit from participation in a Phase II clinical trial is unknown. *Phase III* clinical trials utilize treatments that have evidence of efficacy. These studies examine different dosing regimens and methods of administration of treatment, and they evaluate less common side effects. *Phase IV* clinical trials are conducted on drugs or devices that have been approved by the U.S. Food and Drug Administration to understand how well a treatment works in a broad, heterogenous mix of patients and to gather information about potential side effects.

Participation in clinical trials requires the ability to integrate complex information. People should understand the purpose of the trial, the potential risks and benefits, whether they will be randomly assigned to a treatment condition, when the study will end, and whether they have the right to access the experimental treatment when the study ends. Although the consenting process requires that patients be provided with extensive information about the nature of the research, it is impossible to know the degree to which decisions about participation are influenced by a multitude of factors, including intelligence, emotions, physical illness, interpersonal relationships, and underlying beliefs.

CASE EXAMPLE

June was a 49-year-old woman diagnosed with a ductal carcinoma in situ breast cancer. She underwent treatment that she understood to be curative, but she returned to her surgeon after 2 years with concerns about a painful area that she feared was cancer. She was dismissed and had the perception that her surgeon found her to be a hypochondriac. Her communication style was often tangential, and in therapy it took long periods of uninterrupted time to fully understand her. June made multiple visits to different physician specialties over the following 5 years before she was diagnosed with Stage IV breast cancer. After a genetic mutation was identified the following year, she became eligible for a Phase I clinical trial testing a targeted therapy. She expressed deep regret and anger that her earlier complaints had been dismissed and wished that she had known more about how to advocate for herself. Her trust in the medical profession was diminished. Trial participation required travel out of state. As a single mother, the decision required weighing the hope that her cancer would be responsive to the treatment against the potential time away from her adolescent son and the quality of her remaining time. She was required to discontinue her current treatment to wash out the effects of the drug before starting the clinical trial, and she feared that in so doing, she might die even sooner. Nonetheless, she was optimistic and placed a great deal of faith in the treating physician and the reputation of the cancer center where she was treated. June took little time to decide about participation in the trial, but as she waited the necessary weeks to wash out chemotherapy, she reviewed each element of the decision-making process and sought validation from her other medical specialists, friends, and family and processed the decision in therapy.

June' case underscores that people who decide to participate in clinical trials cite the following reasons: hope for therapeutic benefit (43%), confidence in their physician (30%), and altruistic hope that others might benefit (21%), as well as the feeling that they have no other alternative, that the trial provides the benefit of free care and medication, and trust in the institution and/or influence by family or friends (ECRI Institute, 2002). Ideally, psychosocial oncology care should be available to support patients as they grapple with important medical decisions and the associated emotions.

TWO

PSYCHOLOGICAL ASSESSMENT AND INTERVENTIONS FOR COMMON COMORBID PROBLEMS

Assessment and Treatment
of Depression

Approximately 10% to 17% of patients with cancer have clinically significant symptoms of depression (Linden, Vodermaier, MacKenzie, & Greig, 2012; Ng, Boks, Zainal, & de Wit, 2011; Pinquart & Duberstein, 2010). Depressive symptoms usually peak during treatment and diminish in the year following diagnosis (Krebber et al., 2014). Yet depression often goes undetected and untreated. More than one third of patients with pancreatic cancer are depressed (Massie, 2004). Compared with the general population, the prevalence of clinically significant depressive symptoms is higher in patients with lung (13.0%–17.9%), gynecological (10.9%–16.5%), breast (9.3%–10.7%), and colorectal (7.0%) cancer (Linden et al., 2012; Walker et al., 2014). Estimates of rates of depression in oncology subgroups vary widely because of the wide heterogeneity in measures, time points at which depressive symptoms are assessed, and degree to which comorbid physical illness symptoms are controlled for in the existing literature on

http://dx.doi.org/10.1037/0000054-005
Psychological Treatment of Patients With Cancer, by E. A. Dornelas

this topic. However, similar to many other types of medical illness (e.g., heart disease), depression rates are highest among younger patients with cancer, regardless of other salient disease characteristics.

Risk factors for the development of depression following a cancer diagnosis include prior history of depression, female gender, younger age, distressed relationships or social supports, and greater acuity of illness. Protective factors associated with greater resiliency include good social support, active lifestyle, positive expectations regarding prognosis, problem-focused orientation, and faith in the medical system or physician.

RISKS ASSOCIATED WITH DEPRESSIVE SYMPTOMS

Evidence indicates that untreated depression is associated with disease progression (Lutgendorf, Sood, & Antoni, 2010). Clinically significant depression shortens survival times in patients with breast and lung cancer, leukemia, lymphoma, and brain tumor. A meta-analysis of 76 studies estimates the relative risk of mortality increased by 17% in patients with cancer with depression compared with those without depression (Pinquart & Duberstein, 2010). Depression might affect cancer progression and mortality in a number of ways. Low mood influences health behaviors, such as compliance with medical regimens and motivation to exercise, and often coexists with other health risks, such as alcohol abuse or tobacco use. In addition, people with symptoms of depression can be socially isolated or have conflicted relationships such that they may not have some of the tangible supports (e.g., transportation to medical visits) that affect cancer survival. Health care providers might inadvertently treat patients with depression differently. In a study of 1,868 people with pancreatic cancer, Boyd et al. (2012) found that people with distant disease and depression had lower likelihood of receiving chemotherapy; after adjusting for these factors, depression did not predict survival. Physiologically, depression is associated with inflammation, suppressed immune response, and heightened sympathetic reactivity, all of which are in turn correlated with cancer progression in some, but not all, cases. The many pathways and mechanisms by which depressive symptoms and cancer interact are not yet well understood. From a quality-of-life perspective, it is clear that treating depressed mood is a critical part of cancer care. No conclusive evidence indicates that effective treatment for depression improves cancer survival, but preliminary studies have found that psychological intervention improves overall and cancer-specific mortality (Andersen et al., 2008). This type of research is not easy to conduct, because of the methodological challenges of controlling for the diversity of tumor types, depression measures, and inherent difficulties in delivering psychotherapeutic interventions in a large-scale randomized controlled trial.

DEPRESSION SCREENING

The Commission on Cancer requires that patients with cancer be screened for distress at pivotal points in treatment in order for an institution to be accredited, but the merits of screening specifically for depression continue to be debated. This section focuses on depression; and screening for distress is addressed in Chapter 5. Routine screening would have the potential to identify many more patients who experience treatable symptoms of depression. The nine-item Patient Health Questionnaire (PHQ-9; Spitzer, Kroenke, & Williams, 1999) is a depression screener that was evaluated in a sample of 4,264 patients with cancer. Using a cutoff of ≥ 8, the PHQ-9 showed 93% sensitivity and 81% specificity to detect major depressive disorder in this patient population (Thekkumpurath et al., 2011), and it is a measure with good diagnostic accuracy. Although patients with cancer often have more somatic symptoms (sleep problems, loss of energy) than people without cancer, the single score to screen for depression is preferable to examining the cognitive–affective and somatic items separately. A large study comparing 2,059 people treated for cancer against a representative community sample of 2,693 participants confirmed that the PHQ-9 performs best as a single dimension rather than a two-factor structure. The American Society of Clinical Oncology guidelines recommend screening for depression using the PHQ-9 with the cutoff threshold of ≥ 8 (Andersen et al., 2014). However, opponents of routine screening argue that the understanding of how and when to screen oncology patients for depression is inadequate. A review of 19 studies found no evidence that routine screening for depression improves psychological outcomes over usual care (Meijer et al., 2011). Because psychological treatment resources are limited and disproportionately favor pharmacological intervention over psychotherapy, screening also carries the risk that antidepressants will be increasingly overutilized. Meijer et al. (2011) recommended that randomized controlled trials be conducted to evaluate the benefit of routine screening for depression over usual care.

The PHQ-2 is a two-item subset from the PHQ-9 that measures anhedonia and low mood. A positive score indicates a need for further screening. The PHQ-2 has strong psychometric properties, clearly defined cut points, is specific for depression rather than distress, can be administered by nonmental health professionals, and is not burdensome to patients (Kroenke & Spitzer, 2002). The PHQ-2 has a sensitivity of 93% and specificity of 81% to detect depression in an oncology population (Mitchell, 2008). Patients who are flagged for possible depressed mood benefit from completing the PHQ-9 along with clinical interview.

A substantial number of patients with cancer who screen positive for depression have a prior history of depression and are already on antidepressants and/or in counseling. In such cases, it is important to assess whether the current medication and/or psychotherapy regimen is appropriate and sufficiently intensive.

Often, patients are screened for depression by nursing staff, and further assessment by mental health professionals is warranted. In cases in which behavioral health specialists and counselors are embedded within a cancer treatment center, it can be easier to refer patients for treatment. However, it can be difficult to refer patients with cancer to community therapists if they do not perceive themselves to be distressed or do not see any benefit to counseling. The art of making a referral for mental health is not always well executed in medicine. Many people feel that seeking psychological help is stigmatizing or a sign of weakness. A statement such as the following can be one way to assess a patient's receptiveness to help: "You have been going through a lot since you were diagnosed with cancer. I wonder if it would help to have another person to talk to outside the family, such as psychologist or counselor, who could provide additional support?"

Patients usually understand that they will have a natural psychological adjustment to a cancer diagnosis, but they do not realize that physiological changes that occur as a side effect of some cancer treatments (e.g., hypothyroidism) can trigger depressive episodes. For example, hormone replacement therapy in women with breast cancer triggers hormonal fluctuation that can precipitate or exacerbate depressed mood. Psychologists are often resistant to use of the term *counselor*, appropriately noting that psychological intervention is far broader than counseling. But from a patient perspective, the term *counseling* connotes a more palatable approach and is a benign term that is more easily understood than *behavioral health* and perceived as less stigmatizing compared with terms such as *psychological* or *mental health* treatment.

TREATMENT FOR DEPRESSION

Psychological intervention is effective in treating depression, anxiety, and quality of life in cancer survivors (Osborn, Demoncada, & Feuerstein, 2006). Of the many studies of psychological intervention for oncology patients, only a minority are randomized controlled trials specifically designed for oncology patients with clinical depression and have depression as the primary outcome of interest. A meta-analysis that included six studies of psychotherapeutic treatment for oncology patients who were depressed showed moderate effect sizes for treatment over control (Hart et al., 2012).

Cognitive Behavioral Therapy

A number of evidence-based psychotherapeutic approaches have been shown to be effective in treating patients with cancer with depression, and evidence is strong that cognitive behavioral therapy (CBT) is effective in this regard (Hart et al., 2012). CBT has been shown to have both medium- and long-term benefits in mixed oncology populations. The underlying premise of CBT for depression is that maladaptive cognitions can give rise to depression and distressed mood. Of course, maladaptive cognitions can also trigger anxiety and a host of other psychological responses. The premise of this book is that the reader has a fund of knowledge in standard psychological interventions and the ability to appropriately generalize knowledge across topics covered in each chapter. Hence an in-depth overview of CBT is beyond the scope of this book, but in brief, Beck's (1976) model of CBT is based on the theory that cognitive schemas give rise to distorted automatic thoughts that in turn promulgate emotional distress. Table 4.1 provides examples of cognitive distortions manifested in the context of cancer treatment.

Table 4.1

Examples of Cognitive Reframing in the Context of Cancer Care

Type of cognitive distortion	Example	Cognitive reframing
Catastrophic thinking	I have cancer and am going to die.	It will take time to see how I will respond to treatment.
Disqualifying or minimizing the positive	My doctor says there is no evidence of cancer, but it is just a matter of time.	Although there are no guarantees about the future, having no evidence of cancer is encouraging.
Overgeneralization	My ex-spouse causes me stress, and if my cancer returns, it is his or her fault!	There are no simple reasons why cancer recurs. I'm in control of how I choose to react to stressors.
Emotional reasoning	I feel depressed because I'm so physically sick from chemotherapy.	Feeling sick is a side effect of treatment. Focusing on small moments of pleasure helps.
Personalization	My doctor really doesn't care about me, she or he didn't even personally make the call to give me my test results.	Oncologists are not infallible. I can talk to my doctor about my test results.
Mental filter	Cancer is fed by sugar; if I control my sugar intake, my cancer won't come back.	There is no one simple cause of cancer, and following normal dietary guidelines is the best way to take care of myself.
All-or-nothing thinking	My child is my only priority; I can't worry about my own self-care.	By taking care of myself, I'm helping my child because she or he needs me to be healthy.

A diagnosis of cancer typically stimulates the automatic thought of a foreshortened life. People with no prior medical history are usually shocked to learn they have been diagnosed with cancer. The thought of dying imminently from cancer is realistic for patients with a cancer that is diagnosed at an advanced stage. The majority of patients diagnosed with localized, early-stage cancer are not likely to die prematurely from their disease. It can be difficult to find the balance between being aware that one's lifespan may be foreshortened and remaining focused on life's everyday events. A patient with late-stage pancreatic cancer quoted the character Andy DuFresne from the film *The Shawshank Redemption*: "I guess it comes down to a simple choice, really. Get busy living or get busy dying" (Marvin & Darabout, 1994).

CBT delivered in individual therapy is more effective than group intervention, but both modalities have significant effects. Although many studies testing CBT to treat depressed cancer patients have focused on women with breast cancer, meta-analyses indicate that there is sufficient evidence to conclude that CBT is effective in improving depressive symptoms across many cancer diagnoses and stages of disease (Osborn et al., 2006).

Behavioral activation (Lejuez, Hopko, Acierno, Daughters, & Pagoto, 2011) is an effective component of CBT in treating depressed mood. Evidence indicates that behavioral activation for oncology patients who are depressed has substantial benefit. Steps of a behavioral activation protocol include

- self-monitoring of physical activity,
- identifying the highest priority goals that are most completely aligned with personal values,
- establishing an activity hierarchy of activities ranked from easiest to most difficult, and
- setting weekly goals and logging physical activity.

Behavioral activation could simply refer to performing normal activities of daily living, returning to work or engaging in new activities (e.g., exercise) that were not part of the individual's prior repertoire of skills. Physical activity is effective in treating depressed mood in people with cancer and described in more detail in the following section.

Exercise

The majority of studies of exercise tested in patients with cancer do not specifically target depressive symptoms, and most subjects do not meet criteria for depression. Thus, it is impressive that a meta-analysis (Craft, Vaniterson, Helenowski, Rademaker, & Courneya, 2012) demonstrated that exercise has a modest positive effect on depressive symptoms across a variety of cancer diagnoses, stages, and severity of symptoms. Studies of clinically depressed cancer patients may show even stronger effects for exercise. Exercise programs of at least 30 minutes' duration, that are supervised, and that are not performed at home are associated with strong effect sizes for depression.

A mental health professional is often in a position to recommend exercise and refer to community-based programs with the goal of improved quality of life. One such program is LIVESTRONG at the YMCA, which is based on the principle that exercise in a group setting offers both support from others living with cancer and physical rehabilitation (Heston, Schwartz, Justice-Gardiner, & Hohman, 2015). This 12-week, community-based intervention has been shown to have a positive influence on many domains, including strength, fatigue, insomnia, and perceived social support (Rajotte et al., 2012). People who attend LIVESTRONG at the YMCA state that they find it is helpful to realize that they are not alone and that physical activity can improve their mood and physical well-being. Although physical rehabilitation to regain cardiac and pulmonary functioning is considered the standard of care, oncology has not yet fully tested the efficacy of physical rehabilitation in cancer recovery nor implemented it on a wide-scale basis as part of the routine delivery of care.

HOPELESSNESS AND SUICIDE

Left untreated, depression can be lethal for a minority of patients. The incidence of suicide in people diagnosed with cancer is double that of the general population. One third of suicides in patients with cancer occur within the first 30 days after the initial diagnosis, and risk remains elevated for at least 1 year (Anguiano, Mayer, Piven, & Rosenstein, 2012; Walker et al., 2008) Even among people with curable cancers, rates of suicidal ideation are higher for both men and women. For example, many men survive prostate cancer but have disproportionately higher rates of suicide compared with men with no cancer diagnosis (Misono, Weiss, Fann, Redman, & Yueh, 2008). Site of cancer is associated with increased risk. Patients with cancers of the lung, stomach, oral cavity, pharynx, larynx, and have disproportionately higher incidence of suicide. People are more likely to consider suicide when they have a life-threatening diagnosis; face intractable pain; lose bowel or bladder function; deal with amputation; or cannot speak, eat, or swallow. Some cancer survivors express the wish that they had not survived, because of their diminished quality of life. Symptom management in such patients is critical. Patients who desire to die feel sicker and weaker than others and are more likely to report social isolation and feeling that they are a burden to others. They are also more likely to report loss of dignity, control, anxiety, depression, and hopelessness. However, in studies of patients who state that they want to die, many do not report anxiety or depression; therefore, screening for hopelessness may be more salient in identifying potentially suicidal patients (Rosenfeld et al., 2014).

Suicidal ideation, attempt, or completion may be viewed as a communication of suffering and despair rather than readiness to die. One way to open a conversation about suicide is to state that "many people think about death after a cancer diagnosis." The "Ask Suicide-Screening Questions to Everyone in Medical Settings" project is a federally funded study designed by principal investigator Lisa Horowitz to determine the best method of assessing suicidal ideation in medical inpatients (see https://www.clinicaltrials.gov/ct2/show/NCT02140177). Assessment questions include the following: "In the past month have you thought of suicide?" and "Have you made a suicide attempt in the past?" If the answer to either is yes, the follow-up questions include "Are you having those thoughts right now?" and "Have you thought about how you would do it?" Patients with cancer need a stepped approach to suicide assessment. Screening instruments are only a first step and need to lead to a discussion between a clinician and patient about the causes of their distress and their circumstances.

Many completed suicides are preceded (Misono et al., 2008) by an attempt. The completion rate of suicide among people diagnosed with cancer is 50% higher than the general population (Greenberg, 2011). Although this is a difficult topic to study, research suggests that many suicide attempts in patients with cancer are related to the combination of uncontrolled pain and hopelessness (Klonsky & May, 2015). Collaborative partnerships between oncologists, pain management specialists, and mental health professionals are essential to effectively decrease suffering in patients who are suicidal. Families and clinicians are traumatized in the aftermath of a suicide. Suicide can be stigmatizing for the partner, children, or parents of the patient. In addition, risk of suicide increases with age (Misono et al., 2008). As the U.S. population ages and there are more cancer survivors, it will become even more vital to find effective methods of preventing the physical and emotional suffering that gives rise to suicidal ideation. There is a critical difference between patients who want to die and those who desire medical-aid-in-dying, a topic addressed in Chapter 10.

PATIENT ENGAGEMENT

Depression is often difficult for health care providers, family members, and patients to recognize because its somatic symptoms overlap with the effects of cancer and chemotherapy. Even once depression is acknowledged, patients may not feel confident that psychological intervention could be of value in helping them cope with their illness. Engagement of medical patients into mental health treatment is an understudied topic.

CASE EXAMPLE

Ray was a robust construction worker with advanced colon cancer. In his initial telephone call, he said,

> My doctor recommended that I call, but I'm not sure I need counseling. Am I depressed, of course I'm depressed! Anyone would be depressed with this diagnosis. I'm not sure what a therapist could do for me and I don't really want any more medical appointments. (He acknowledged that he had never sought any mental health treatment over his lifetime.)

Over the phone, the therapist suggested that it is often easier to talk with someone other than close family when dealing with life-threatening illness:

> I might suggest going for a consultation, then making the decision about whether counseling could be of any help. The worst-case scenario: You waste an hour of your time. The best outcome: you feel better than you do at present and are at your best to cope with everything that is going on.

By making the appointment personally and clarifying that no commitment to therapy was expected, the therapist created an initial rapport and alleviated the patient's fears about committing to ongoing treatment. People feel less resistant to an initial consultation when they understand that decisions are within their control. It is important to ensure that the initial consultation elicits a sense of hope and provides a clear framework of how the therapist can be helpful. If the initial consultation is devoted simply to assessment, patients who are naive to mental health treatment often see no value and are unlikely to return. Questions about early developmental history are usually not viewed as germane to the presenting problem by the patient. In this regard, initial psychotherapy assessments in the field of clinical health psychology usually need to forgo extensive information gathering about historical data and focus primarily on the reason for the referral. Should the patient engage in treatment, other pertinent history can be gathered in subsequent patient encounters.

Accessibility plays a critical role in seeking treatment. Ideally, psychological services are colocated within the cancer center or treatment facility. Therapists who book their own appointments (rather than relying on administrative assistants) can answer questions or allay fears about what will be involved in treatment. Specific training in working with people with cancer and referral from a trusted oncologist are important factors that contribute to the perceived credibility of the behavioral health specialist. Psychological intervention is still associated with stigma. Normalizing depressed mood as a common part of the cancer experience helps reduce reluctance to seek or accept mental health treatment. A multidisciplinary team that includes providers who can assess, deliver psychotherapeutic intervention, prescribe psychotropic medications, and assist with accessing necessary social services is ideal, although such a team is rarely fully accessible in most American health care systems. The majority of oncology patients who are moderately depressed are untreated or undertreated, causing unnecessary suffering and placing greater burden on medical providers of oncology care.

INTEGRATED CARE

Despite the fact that psychological intervention is underutilized for oncology patients who are distressed, existing providers are typically inundated with referrals. It is a complex task to navigate mental health treatment. It is thus not surprising that many medical professionals have little understanding of how to match the patient with the right level and type of mental health treatment. A guide to local psychiatric and psychological services in the community is very useful and can be developed by the mental health professional who has more knowledge in this area. Oncology nurses can provide a warm handoff to behavioral health specialists.

It is the norm, not the exception, that people with depression and cancer have a variety of other life circumstances that contribute to their depression (e.g., distress related to their marriage, children, or work). The mental health provider embedded in a cancer center who attempts to work long-term on issues unrelated to cancer will quickly reach full capacity with no bandwidth to address the needs of constant patient turnover. It is critical to identify the parameters of treatment, discuss the treatment model, and obtain a priori agreement about the types of issues that will be worked on and a general idea of the time frame. Patients with a strong sense of loss in terminating treatment or transitioning to a community provider can elicit feelings of guilt and countertransference from the clinician. Independent practitioners working in the community are different from hospital-based providers in that they can more easily accommodate open-ended therapy and thus tailor the treatment to the patient's needs.

CULTURAL ISSUES

Ethnic identity and socioeconomic status influence both perceptions of depression and treatment seeking. Racial and ethnic minorities, people who are impoverished, and those who are non-English speakers are not well represented in large-scale clinical trials testing treatments for depression. A small study of 74 patients with cancer compared African Americans with and without depression versus Whites with depression. African American patients with cancer who were depressed were more likely to endorse symptoms such as irritability, insomnia, and fatigue, as well as social isolation compared with Whites (Zhang, Gary, & Zhu, 2015). In the largest study to date of depression and anxiety in the Hispanic and Latino population, Wassertheil-Smoller et al. (2014) found that 27% of 16,000 adult respondents reported high levels of depressive symptoms, but only 5% received antidepressant treatment. Although this study did not focus specifically on oncology patients, it is noteworthy for its size and its inclusion of large groups of Mexicans, Cubans, Dominicans, Puerto Ricans, and Central and South Americans from New York, Miami, San Diego, and Chicago. More than one third (38%) of Puerto Rican respondents endorsed high levels of depression, compared with 22% of Mexicans. Importantly, first- and second-generation Latinos were more likely to report high levels of depressive symptoms than were those born in other countries (Wassertheil-Smoller et al., 2014). Similarly, Asian Americans are a highly diverse subgroup in the United States who are underdiagnosed and undertreated for depression. Asian American women age 65 and older have higher rates of suicide compared with any other ethnic or racial subgroup in the United States (Yeung & Kam, 2006). Chinese Americans are more likely to endorse somatic rather than affective symptoms of depression and less likely to consider themselves depressed. Asian Americans are more likely to associate mental health treatment with stigma. Some Chinese Americans are more comfortable with traditional Chinese medicine, such as acupuncture, meditation, or tai chi, than with psychotherapy. Chinese medicine also has an entire herbal armamentarium to help patients balance the yin yang of their qi. More research about depression in racial and ethnic subgroups is needed. The potential for misunderstanding in the psychotherapeutic process is high, as is the need for more in-depth cultural sensitivity training for mental health clinicians.

SUMMARY

The consequences of untreated depression can be lethal and, minimally, interfere with quality of life. Some people suffering from depression may be more receptive to treatment in the context of a cancer diagnosis. Evidence-based treatments that are effective for the treatment of depression in the general population (e.g., CBT, exercise, behavioral activation) are also effective in the oncology population and should be integrated into the routine delivery of care.

5

Assessment and Treatment of Anxiety

Anxiety is a normal reaction to a frightening diagnosis. A substantial number of people develop clinically significant anxiety during and after cancer treatment, and a subset of patients develop phobias or post-traumatic stress disorder (PTSD). On average, about one of 10 people diagnosed with cancer meet clinical criteria for anxiety in studies in which interview methods were used to establish the diagnosis (Mitchell, Ferguson, Gill, Paul, & Symonds, 2013). Prevalence of specific phobia in patients with cancer has been estimated to be 13% (Stark et al., 2002). In addition, family members and caregivers of patients with cancer experience high levels of distress and anxiety (Mitchell et al., 2013).

Cancer increases risk for symptoms of acute stress disorder and cancer-related PTSD. However, it is very difficult to gauge the prevalence of PTSD and acute stress disorder in people with cancer, particularly

http://dx.doi.org/10.1037/0000054-006
Psychological Treatment of Patients With Cancer, by E. A. Dornelas

because the *Diagnostic and Statistical Manual of Mental Disorders* (5th ed.; *DSM–5*; American Psychiatric Association, 2013) recently revised the symptom clusters that define PTSD. Symptoms such as avoidance, hyperarousal, and intrusive reexperiencing are commonly reported in clinical psychosocial oncology practice. It is important to be cautious about making broad generalizations about anxiety in people because it is operationally defined in a variety of ways across studies and is influenced by many factors. The continuum of reaction ranges from typical to more extreme presentations of preexisting or new anxiety disorders.

FACTORS RELATED TO ANXIETY

Although anxiety is a typical adjustment reaction to a diagnosis of cancer, it can be exacerbated if the patient experiences symptoms or treatments that are frightening or cause physiological arousal, such as rapid heart rate. For example, patients with lung cancer often experience dyspnea (difficulty breathing), which in turn can trigger anxiety. Anxiety can be experienced as a side effect of certain medications (e.g., corticosteroids). A variety of factors, including severity of illness, age, level of pain, fatigue, history of anxiety, living alone, and personal experience with a friend or family member's experience of cancer, influence the likelihood of experiencing anxiety.

Cognitive factors, such as perceptions, beliefs, and attitudes about cancer, affect a person's ability to cope with their cancer-related anxiety. Most people are not able to accurately predict their risk of cancer recurrence. In a study about accuracy of perceived risk in more than 500 patients with breast cancer, women with less social support and more anxiety, and those diagnosed with ductal carcinoma in situ (DCIS), were likely to overestimate their risk, and non-White women were more likely to underestimate their risk (Liu et al., 2010). Anxiety is the most consistent and strongest predictor of overestimation of breast cancer risk (Partridge et al., 2008). Counseling about actual risk has not been shown to improve accuracy of risk perception (Lerman et al., 1995). The problem is important because evidence suggests that high levels of anxiety influence decisions about medical treatment. For example, men with early-stage prostate cancer and high anxiety levels are more likely to choose aggressive treatment rather than surveillance (Latini et al., 2007).

TRAJECTORY OF ANXIETY

Anxiety is typically high immediately following diagnosis, peaks at time of surgery, and remains elevated for about 1 year. When people end active cancer treatment, their anxiety often increases. Patients often report that they felt more secure when they were seeing their oncologist frequently. Nearly 18% of cancer survivors report persistent anxiety 2 years to 10 years posttreatment (Mitchell et al., 2013). Many patients express concern that imaging and testing is not part of their follow-up treatment plan. The *National Comprehensive Cancer Network Clinical Practice Guidelines in Oncology* (see https://www.nccn.org/professionals/physician_gls/f_guidelines.asp) do not recommend routine imaging or testing as part of long-term surveillance for many subgroups of patients with cancer because no evidence indicates that such testing improves overall or disease-free survival. Many cancer survivors feel uneasy waiting to see if and when symptoms recur. It is difficult for a layperson to interpret whether a symptom warrants visiting the oncologist. Nonrelated symptoms (e.g., headache) can trigger worry that cancer has recurred in the form of a brain tumor. On the other end of the spectrum, patients who undergo routine scans, track biomarkers, or have other diagnostic tests as part of their follow-up surveillance describe an emotional rollercoaster, characterized by high levels of anxiety in the period of time leading up to diagnostic tests or procedures and great relief for a period of time upon getting news of no sign of recurrence or progression. Anxiety and distress ratchet up when cancer recur or progresses, as they do during periods of exacerbation, such as hospitalization.

COPING WITH CANCER

People resort to their own unique, default adaptive or maladaptive coping strategies to deal with cancer. Maladaptive coping strategies include substance abuse and extreme forms of denial, such as avoiding necessary cancer treatment, dissociation, and intellectualization.

Case Example

A patient with some limited medical background, diagnosed with an aggressive Stage IV lung cancer, was referred for counseling. He was taking long periods of time to debate whether the proper testing had been done and questioned whether the diagnosis was accurate. There had been an error in the tests ordered at another institution, and the patient viewed this as evidence that the diagnosis could be incorrect. However, his physicians and a nationally known oncologist sought for a second opinion were unanimous in their recommendation to seek treatment quickly. Treatment was delayed by months as he requested copies of all of his medical records and struggled to understand the implications. His radiation oncologist was unable to persuade him to begin treatment and angered him when she suggested that he might be anxious. The patient was not in agreement to seek counseling but agreed to come to one session.

At the session, he presented with a long and detailed explanation of his understanding of his medical diagnosis but expressed that he had substantial concern that he might be wrongly diagnosed. His affect was flat, and he noted that he saw no value in getting emotional, particularly because he felt it was important that he spend his time doing research to confirm the validity of his diagnosis. He used the Internet to research unfamiliar terms that he came across when reviewing his medical records. He did not see himself as anxious.

The therapist used a problem-solving approach to elicit the patient's perceptions of the pros and cons of delaying treatment. The therapist was empathetic to the patient's logic and explored whether he felt trusting of his primary oncologist, and he acknowledged that he felt it was critical that he place trust in his physician. The patient did not return for counseling for several months after the first session but did undergo recommended treatment. He returned for treatment after 2 months because his medical oncologist suggested he might be anxious. The patient emphasized that his anxiety was highly appropriate to his diagnosis. He still felt some residual doubt as to the validity of the diagnosis and hoped that it would be proved to be incorrect. He also noted that he had quit smoking more than 10 years ago but now experienced deep feelings of regret that he had not stopped sooner. He questioned whether medical professionals judged him for having smoked. He showed much greater range of affect compared with his first session. He said that he agreed to come back because he felt that a concrete suggestion from the therapist had been helpful. The therapist had suggested that he shift gears from his medical research to identify something each day to take pleasure in, whether it was big or small. He said that shifting his focus to spending less time on the Internet researching his disease and much more time focused on pleasurable activities had been helpful. In his first session, he had come across as brittle and highly defended. After having time to adjust to the diagnosis and treatment, he appeared more resilient and showed greater willingness to recognize and express his emotions.

This illustrative case underscores that an unexpected stressor, such as a diagnosis of terminal illness, is a shock that can easily trigger maladaptive responses, regardless of how bright or high functioning the person might be. The patient utilized problem-focused coping strategies of seeking information and taking control and responded well to the problem-solving approach of evaluating the pros and cons of delaying treatment to conduct more of his own research. *Emotion-focused coping* refers to methods of managing the affective states that influence perception of a stressor. People who make an active effort to acknowledge, process, and express their feelings about cancer tend to experience less distress over time (Stanton et al., 2000). Emotion-focused coping can help a person to clarify their values and reach greater clarity about how they want to spend their time and energy. Expression of emotion also can help people to connect with important family members or friends and feel supported and is associated with longer survival in women with breast cancer (Reynolds et al., 2000).

The patient described in the example above is noteworthy for the intensity and persistence of his denial. Denial is a psychological defense or coping strategy that ranges on a continuum from helpful to harmful. Although the tendency to minimize attention to stressors can be quite healthy, at the other end of the spectrum, an unwillingness to entertain the possibility of a cancer diagnosis or need for treatment is fraught with risk. In the last months of life, denial is normative and might be an unconscious method of protecting the self from emotions that are too overwhelming or difficult to bear.

MINDFULNESS AND HOPE

Mindfulness-based stress reduction (MBSR) is an evidence-based clinical approach to helping people with newly diagnosed and recurrent cancer to feel more engaged with life. Although prior research has shown that supportive–expressive therapy has benefits for people with cancer (Spiegel, Kraemer, Bloom, & Gottheil, 1989), recent research has studied interventions focused on mindfulness and hope. *Mindfulness* refers to the basic principle that people should live in the moment. It focuses not on trying to change negative emotions but on simply accepting them. Meditative techniques are used to gain the ability to maintain awareness of the present moment as well as an open and curious state of mind. MBSR is most often delivered as an intensive, group program lasting about 8 weeks, with weekly meditation and an all-day silent retreat. Participants practice sitting meditation, walking meditation, hatha yoga, and body scan. Variations of this approach have been tested in multiple studies of patients with cancer, with support for MBSR's effectiveness in reducing anxiety and depression in patients with breast cancer (Cramer, Lauche, Paul, & Dobos, 2012). This type of intensive intervention is acceptable only to a subset of patients with cancer but learning techniques to maintain mindfulness is helpful in diminishing cancer-related anxiety.

Hope therapy is based on the construct that hope reflects a person's motivation and capacity to work toward personally salient goals (Snyder, Rand, & Sigmon, 2002). *Hope* in this context refers to the belief in one's ability to make new goals and work toward them. The construct has face validity, with evidence indicating that psychological intervention aimed at eliciting hope is effective at increasing hope and reducing distress in women with breast cancer (Rustøen, Cooper, & Miaskowski, 2011; Thornton et al., 2014). However, a meta-analysis of hope therapy that included 27 studies in community settings (albeit with small sample sizes) found no effect for hope therapy on psychological distress (Weis & Speridakos, 2011). The authors concluded that results of the meta-analysis suggest the need to refine the theoretical model. Only four of the 27 studies were focused on people with cancer. The other 23 studies had diverse samples that included high school and college students, incarcerated women, psychiatric outpatients, and nursing home residents. It is possible that as more studies are published, meta-analyses focused on oncology samples might yield different results. The goals of hope therapy are consistent with a psychotherapeutic approach aimed not at eradicating worry but instead at learning to cope more successfully with anxiety and to shift energy into personally meaningful pursuits.

ANXIETY IN THE CONTEXT OF EARLY STAGE CANCER

There has been a dramatic shift in the United States toward screening and early detection of the most common cancers: breast, prostate, and colorectal. To that end, the numbers of women diagnosed with DCIS and men diagnosed with prostate cancer have increased dramatically. Welch, Schwartz, and Woloshin (2011) noted that mammogram and prostate-specific antigen testing have high false-positive rates that can result in unnecessary treatment, as well as anxiety. A diagnosis of a cancer that is indolent or curable still generates considerable anxiety, even when people are given factual information about their risk. More than one of four women diagnosed with DCIS have highly overinflated risk perceptions (Partridge et al., 2008). Why do people persist in incorrect beliefs about their risk? The emotional impact of a cancer diagnosis is so profound that it may be difficult to assimilate new information about risk status. Perhaps by continuing to overinflate risk, people prepare themselves for negative outcomes. It is important to note that patient perceptions also reflect differences of opinions among medical professionals. Partridge et al. (2008) found that 40% of physicians surveyed "always" refer to DCIS as cancer, whereas 22% "never" refer to DCIS as cancer. However, high anxiety is the most important predictor of fear of recurrence. Women with high anxiety levels are 4 times more likely to substantially overestimate their risk of recurrence compared with those who are not anxious. Most commonly, people report intrusive thoughts and fears about symptoms. Psychological intervention with patients who have been diagnosed with early-stage cancers is easier when the patient's medical oncologist provides history and prognostic information. Patient self-report may be unconsciously skewed, and the mental health provider should corroborate with the physician whenever possible to ascertain the reality of the patient's risk. Clinical focus usually relies on helping the patient to shift perception to allow that despite the fact of some risk, "red alert" hypervigilance is harmful to quality of life and of little value in terms of protection from recurrence. Although heightened anxiety in fact compromises health in terms of its impact on immune and metabolic functioning, this information only makes the anxious patient more fearful that stress will indeed cause their cancer to return. To accept that cancer recurrence in early-stage cancers is largely uncontrollable and unpredictable, people with high anxiety need to learn to reappraise their situation realistically and find strategies to divert their thinking when it takes a dangerous turn to the worst-case scenario.

ANXIETY IN THE CONTEXT OF ADVANCED CANCER

Anxiety in the context of advanced cancer is a complex phenomenon to assess and treat. Progression of disease may be accompanied by pain, fatigue, functional impairment, and other distressing symptoms. People with advanced disease have realistic concerns and fears. Greer, Park, Prigerson, and Safren (2010) described a brief protocol that tailors cognitive behavioral therapy to the treatment of anxiety in patients with advanced cancer. The modules include psychoeducation, relaxation training, cognitive therapy to cope with cancer fears, and activity planning. An algorithm for distinguishing worry from realistic fear is described in Figure 5.1.

A mental health professional who helps an anxious patient to gain perspective about their situation can provide much needed comfort. Anxiety and distress are human reactions to cancer. Too often, anxiety is manifested in the context of cancer treatment, but behavioral health treatment is underutilized. Early identification and treatment of anxiety would improve quality of life for patients and oncology health care providers alike.

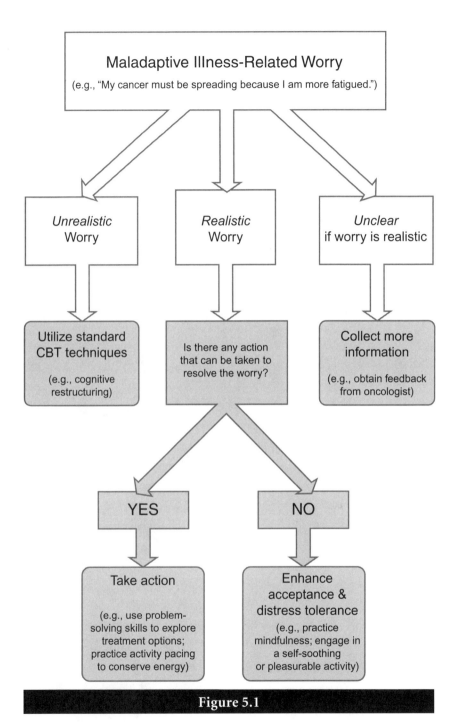

Figure 5.1

CBT algorithm for addressing illness-related worry. From *Avoiding Treatment Failures in the Anxiety Disorders* (p. 319), by M. W. Otto and S. G. Hofmann (Eds.), 2010, New York, NY: Springer. Copyright 2010 by Springer. Reprinted with permission.

6

Sleep Dysregulation and Fatigue

S leep dysregulation and fatigue are by-products of cancer and its treatment. Clinicians are frequently underinformed about how to assess
and treat sleep disturbance and fatigue in this population. Consequently,
behavioral and psychological approaches, although effective, are underutilized. Physicians themselves often do not get enough sleep (ScienceDaily,
2008), and recommendations for the general population are not uniformly
accepted. The National Sleep Foundation (2015) recommends that adults
ages 26 to 64 years sleep 7–9 hours a night and that those over the age of
65 years sleep 7–8 hours a night. The average American, however, sleeps
6.8 hours per night, and 40% get less than the recommended amount of
sleep, according to a 2013 Gallup poll (Jones, 2013).

The methods and measures used to operationalize sleep dysregulation
and fatigue are inconsistent across empirical studies. Some background
and terminology relevant to this literature is reviewed next. Circadian

http://dx.doi.org/10.1037/0000054-007
Psychological Treatment of Patients With Cancer, by E. A. Dornelas
Copyright © 2018 by the American Psychological Association. All rights reserved.

rhythms are biological rhythms that reflect the adaptation of all living things to the rotation of the earth. Circadian rhythms are noted in the migration and hibernation patterns of many species. In humans, the suprachiasmatic nucleus (located in the hypothalamus) is the biological clock that controls biological rhythms, such as core body temperature, fluctuating hormone levels, the menstrual cycle, and sleep–wake patterns. Some tumor types even undergo cell division with greater frequency during specific points during the day (Vanderbilt University, 2010).

Sleep follows a cyclical pattern. A typical sleep cycle lasts approximately 90 minutes and includes both rapid eye movement (REM) and non-REM (NREM) sleep. NREM sleep has four distinct and progressively deeper stages and is characterized by changes in brain wave patterns. REM is the last stage of the sleep cycle; during this stage, the highest brain activity and dreaming are experienced. *Total sleep time* is the sum of both REM and NREM sleep. *Sleep efficiency* is the ratio of the total sleep time to the total time where sleep was potentially possible.

Cancer treatment negatively affects established, synchronized patterns of sleep. Common symptoms reported by people with cancer include fatigue, insomnia, difficulty concentrating, irritability, low energy, and anxiety. This confluence of overlapping symptoms makes it challenging to determine whether sleep disturbance and fatigue symptoms are primarily caused by a primary sleep disorder, one or more mental health conditions, cancer treatment, the cancer itself, or a situational reaction to stressors, although these factors all interact and exacerbate each other.

Approximately one third to one half of patients with newly diagnosed cancer and recently treated patients with cancer report sleep problems (Savard, Simard, Blanchet, Ivers, & Morin, 2001). However, it is not possible to know the true prevalence of sleep disorders within cancer diagnoses because of the variability in how sleep disturbance is defined and the heterogeneity within cancer diagnostic subgroups (Otte et al., 2015). The *Diagnostic and Statistical Manual of Mental Health Disorders* (5th ed.; *DSM–5*) revised its section on sleep–wake disorders and contains 10 groups of sleep–wake disorders: (a) insomnia disorder, (b) hypersomnolence disorder, (c) narcolepsy, (d) breathing-related sleep disorders, (e) circadian rhythm sleep disorders, (f) NREM sleep arousal disorders, (g) nightmare disorder, (h) REM sleep behavior disorder, (i) restless legs syndrome, and (j) substance- or medication-induced sleep disorder. This chapter covers the most commonly encountered of these disorders in people with cancer, as well as the phenomenon of cancer-related fatigue.

Cancer-related fatigue is widely recognized in oncology but is not a disorder that exists as such in the *DSM–5*. It is different from sleepiness in that it is a feeling of exhaustion, low energy, and/or asthenia that does not improve with sufficient rest and is higher than would be expected in relation to the amount of physical exertion. The majority (up to 75%) of people undergoing chemotherapy or radiation treatment report some level of fatigue (Prue, Rankin, Allen, Gracey, & Cramp, 2006). Cancer-related fatigue is complicated to study because of the trajectory of fatigue in cancer, which varies according to many factors, including treatment cycle and regimen. Fatigue is subjective; typically fluctuates during cancer treatment; and for many people, persists long after active treatment has ended. Fatigue is common following surgery. During cyclic chemotherapy, fatigue (similar to other side effects) peaks 1–3 days after treatment and then subsides. However, some types of chemotherapy and radiation treatment have cumulative effects; in these cases, fatigue is more likely to increase in severity over the course of treatment. *Chronotherapy* refers to timing the administration of chemotherapy during the circadian cycle that are less likely to create side effects, such as disturbed sleep, but that are most likely to maximize therapeutic effectiveness. Psychological and behavioral interventions may be aimed at the fatigue that is expected with treatment and/or reducing baseline levels of fatigue.

ASSESSMENT

Memory of sleep disturbance and fatigue symptoms over a period of time is very difficult. The best low-cost method of assessment involves asking patients to track their sleep patterns and/or fatigue symptoms objectively using a diary rather than to rely on their recall. Although not always practical, completion of a sleep and activity diary provides extremely useful information to the clinician. It is possible for patients to evaluate their own sleep/wake activity with motion-sensitive trackers now commonly found on smartphones and other devices. These devices make sleep and activity data easily accessible to the patient and clinician. Although not superior to polysomnography, the accuracy of such devices is excellent. It is important to assess the onset and duration of symptoms, as well as the degree to which symptoms interfere with functioning.

Mental health clinicians may not have access to key medical information, nor are they expected to have the foundation of oncology knowledge needed to understand all of the potential contributors to a sleep problem. When possible, it is ideal to get input from the treating physician about the degree to which sleep and fatigue symptoms would be expected as a result of the cancer, its treatment, or other comorbid health conditions. Although it is understandable that patients with cancer who have sleep problems often wish for a single causal factor to be identified that will explain their symptoms, rarely is the etiology single and easily identifiable. Psychoeducation about sleep disturbance and fatigue during cancer treatment is thus usually a critical aspect of the initial interview.

INSOMNIA

Insomnia is an umbrella term that includes difficulty falling asleep, staying asleep, waking too early, and fragmented sleep, with subtypes of insomnia within this broader category. Clinically significant insomnia results in difficulty maintaining daily functioning and can be episodic or persistent. To meet criteria for insomnia, the sleep dysregulation must occur at least 3 nights a week for at least 3 months, without another sleep disorder present, and not be explained by other psychiatric or medical problems. Approximately half of people treated for cancer report insomnia, compared with about 20% of the general population (Prue et al., 2006). Insomnia increases risk for mental health conditions, such as anxiety and depression, but it also is a symptom of these disorders. Insomnia can cause weakened immune functioning, poor cognitive functioning, reduced productivity at work, and serious impairments with tragic consequences (e.g., motor vehicle accidents).

People with advanced cancer sometimes wake with a feeling of suffocation and inability to breathe, which may be due to effects of the disease or treatment, sleep apnea, psychological distress, or some combination of similar factors. Left untreated, this can easily worsen with onsets of acute anxiety and panic during sleep cycles. Patients often report the fear that they will die in their sleep and as a result feel afraid to go to sleep. Regardless of the cause, a cognitive behavioral approach to the treatment of insomnia is effective and is described in more detail in the following section.

COGNITIVE BEHAVIORAL THERAPY FOR SLEEP DYSREGULATION

Strong evidence indicates that CBT is effective in treating sleep dysregulation in patients with cancer (Garland et al., 2014). CBT for sleep dysregulation incorporates five domains: stimulus control, sleep hygiene, sleep restriction, relaxation, and cognitive restructuring.

Stimulus control refers to the focus on associating the bed with sleep. To associate the stimulus, sleep should occur only in bed and nonsleep behaviors (e.g., watching TV, talking on the phone, working on the computer) should not.

Sleep hygiene is the practice of good sleep habits and practices, such as keeping the room cool and maintaining a routine. Sleep hygiene also involves attention to diet (e.g., avoiding caffeine and alcohol, eating a high-fiber diet, getting more fluids during the day, eating high-protein snacks 2 hours before bedtime).

Cognitive restructuring is aimed at addressing the maladaptive automatic thoughts that people experience about trying to fall asleep and the internal monologue that occurs upon waking during the night. Negative, exaggerated thoughts—such as "I won't be able to function tomorrow," "The stress of not sleeping will make my cancer worse," and "I'm overwhelmed by all that I face tomorrow"—are thoughts that are understandable but exacerbate insomnia. To benefit from cognitive restructuring, the patient needs some explanation of the cognitive behavioral model. Taking note of the thoughts and associated emotions is an essential first step in restructuring. Ideally the patient (not the therapist) is the best person to challenge their own thoughts and readjust to more accurate expectations or beliefs. Adaptive thoughts that replace the distorted thought might include "I am probably sleeping more than I realize"; "I may not be at my best, but I'll be able to function tomorrow"; "My cancer will not be affected by a single night with less than optimal sleep"; and "I am capable of tackling one thing at a time tomorrow." Some people with advanced cancer may express the fear that they will die in their sleep, and exploration of that fear can attenuate anxiety.

It is not surprising that people with cancer often find themselves preoccupied with thinking about the disease at night, a time of fewer distraction when fears can be amplified and perspective can be lost—situations tend to look bleaker at 3:00 a.m. than during the day! Cancer can trigger cognitive distortions, warped inferences, and catastrophic thinking in nearly anyone. Helping a patient realize that they are more likely to envision worst-case scenarios at night is essential to developing skills in correcting cognitive distortions that ratchet up anxiety.

Image rehearsal therapy is a cognitively based treatment that improves nightmares. The patient is instructed to write down what they remember about the nightmare but to change aspects of the dream or its ending to override the original disturbing content. Mental rehearsal of the dream for 10 to 20 minutes a day helps to provide reinforcement. Image rehearsal therapy has been endorsed as a best practice for the treatment of nightmares in the general population (Aurora et al., 2010). Studies of image rehearsal therapy in cancer populations are encouraging, and patients report less distress and a greater feeling of empowerment over nightmares (Wellisch & Cohen, 2011).

Relaxation training is beneficial for people who experience dyspnea (breathlessness) and those who are using machines to help them breathe. This is particularly common in patients who have lung, head, and neck cancers. Practice of diaphragmatic breathing for at least 15 minutes/day increases the likelihood that an individual will be able to invoke this skill when they are trying to fall asleep. Guided imagery and self-hypnosis can be learned to induce a state of relaxation. Relaxation training is likely most effective when deployed as part of a combination of therapies (e.g., sleep restriction, sleep hygiene, stimulus control) to improve sleep quality in patients with cancer (Kaplow, 2005).

CANCER-RELATED FATIGUE

Cancer-related fatigue is common and usually increases over time during active treatment. Nearly one third of people with cancer in remission or who are disease free report persistent fatigue more than 1 year after treatment has ended (Bower et al., 2014). Unlike exhaustion caused by lack of sleep, cancer-related fatigue is not caused by overexhaustion and does not remit after rest. People with cancer-related fatigue may state that they have low energy, cannot perform typical daily functions, and lack a sense of vitality. Some factors that may contribute to fatigue include the effect of the cancer, its treatment, nutritional deficits, physical deconditioning and ability to function. It can be difficult for the mental health provider to distinguish between symptoms of depression and cancer-related fatigue, because of the considerable overlap in symptoms. Indeed, history of depressive disorder is a risk factor for cancer-related fatigue and shares the common denominator of inflammation playing a potentially causal role. The American Society of Clinical Oncology guidelines (Bower et al., 2014) for assessing fatigue include the recommendation that the patient rate the fatigue on a scale from 0 to 10, with 0 indicating absence of fatigue and 10 representing the worst imaginable fatigue. Review of the onset, pattern, and duration of fatigue, as well as the factors that alleviate or exacerbate symptoms, is part of a comprehensive assessment. Cancer-related fatigue is still not well understood, but effective treatment is typically multimodal. Exercise is one component that is well established to have benefit for people who have cancer that is in remission and those who are disease free.

EXERCISE

Exercise is underused as a treatment for sleep dysregulation and fatigue in the cancer population and often may seem counterintuitive for the patient. Yet exercise prescriptions to walk each day are highly effective for people with a variety of cancer types (Chiu, Huang, Chen, Hou, & Tsai, 2015). Physical activity can resynchronize rest/activity patterns. Outdoor walking exposes people to sunlight, which is associated with greater levels of daytime alertness. Physical activity that includes stretching, flexibility and strength conditioning is effective in reducing fatigue (Cantarero-Villanueva et al., 2012). People with cancer who establish or maintain patterns of regular physical activity report higher levels of vitality and energy. In general, it is best to avoid exercising within 3 hours of bedtime, but habitual exercise is associated with better sleep. Self-paced walking three to four times a week is associated with improvements in sleep disturbance and fatigue.

ENERGY CONSERVATION AND ACTIVITY MANAGEMENT (ECAM) FOR FATIGUE

Although exercise is contraindicated for many patients with cancer, there is always an optimal zone of activity. Underactivity and overactivity can both lead to fatigue. Although it might seem intuitive that a person with cancer should not deplete their energy on tasks and activities that are not necessarily meaningful or important to them, most people try to keep functioning in their normal day-to-day routine. Education with the patient to evaluate their daily tasks and activities with a goal of priority setting makes a great deal of common sense. Delegating when possible and pacing to take advantage of times of peak energy help are ways to help people successfully direct their energy to key activities. A three-session ECAM intervention for patients in active chemotherapy or radiation treatment delivered over the telephone by research nurses was tested by Barsevick et al. (2004). The control condition consisted of information about nutrition. During Week 1, patients tracked their typical daily activities and sleep and prioritized each activity. This information was reported in the second telephone session, and the intervention focused on creating an energy conservation plan for the week ahead. The last session was devoted to evaluating and refining the plan. The ECAM intervention was associated with reductions in fatigue but not functional improvement.

MASSAGE

Existing studies examining the efficacy of massage to treat cancer-related fatigue are few, but those that exist are promising (Greenlee et al., 2014). Studies of massage therapy are often difficult to conduct due to the difficulty in finding appropriate control groups. A study of patients with breast cancer comparing massage to a light touch comparison group found that weekly Swedish massage was associated with positive response in multiple markers of stress and immune functioning and that these changes persisted over multiple days (Rapaport, Schettler, & Bresee, 2012). Massage can relieve pain, promote healing, reduce anxiety and induce relaxation; thus, it is a viable and accessible intervention for patients with sleep difficulties. Massage is available in many cancer centers but is often underutilized. Massage as part of a multimodal approach to sleep improvement has been shown to have strong effects in reducing cancer-related fatigue and sleep disturbance.

VITALITY

Vitality is a state of feeling energized, rested, motivated and able to pursue life with vigor. It is a distinct factor and subcomponent of psychological well-being (Grossi et al., 2006). Increasing psychological vitality is a goal of behavioral intervention for fatigue in the oncology population. One approach is to ask the patient to identify a period in life when they felt most vital. Eliciting from the patient a decision to partner with the therapist to restore the patient to that level of vitality accomplishes several therapeutic objectives. It provides a clear and personally relevant goal for therapy, deepens rapport, and increases both motivation and confidence. Research suggests that positive expectations about the future are mediated by vitality to promote both mental and physical energy to engage in adaptive behaviors (Hirsch, Molnar, Chang, & Sirois, 2015). Vitality is a strong predictor of weight loss in healthy adults (Swencionis et al., 2013), and further research exploring this factor as it relates to fatigue and sleep problems in people with cancer is warranted.

Most mental health professionals who treat oncology patients are not sleep experts, but the majority of people with cancer who present for psychological treatment have symptoms of sleep dysregulation and/or fatigue. It is helpful to have some understanding of the literature relevant to the topic when doing clinical work with this population.

7

Sexual Dysfunction and Negative Body Image

Many cancer treatments have a substantial negative impact on sexual function. During medical encounters, this important topic is often inadequately discussed. Sexuality is a complicated, multidimensional construct, with much still to be learned about typical sexual functioning in healthy people without cancer. The literature about sexual function across the broad spectrum of cancers is limited. The two most common cancers, breast and prostate, are sex specific, although in rare cases breast cancer also occurs in men. Erectile dysfunction is the most common presentation of sexual side effects in men with prostate cancer. Erectile dysfunction is the norm, rather than the exception for men who have undergone radical prostatectomy and external beam radiation therapy. About half of women who have undergone treatment for breast or gynecological treatment report persisting sexual difficulties (Maiorino, Chiodini, Bellastella, Giugliano, & Esposito, 2016). Approximately 40% of men who have been successfully

http://dx.doi.org/10.1037/0000054-008
Psychological Treatment of Patients With Cancer, by E. A. Dornelas

treated for testicular cancer have persistent erectile dysfunction (Wiechno, Demkow, Kubiak, Sadowska, & Kaminska, 2007). The prevalence of clinically significant sexual side effects in people with other types of cancer varies widely depending on many factors, including the domain of sexual functioning that is assessed, extent of surgical intervention, age, relational quality, comorbid psychiatric conditions, and severity of illness. Research in this field is usually based on self-report and presurgical assessment of sexual functioning is rare. Thus, it is somewhat difficult to evaluate the trajectory of sexual dysfunction prior to, during, and following cancer treatment because the topic is sensitive and few data sources are available.

Loss of desire, loss of sensation, and inability to reach orgasm are distressing side effects of cancer treatment that often do not fully remit after treatment has ended. Dyspareunia (painful intercourse) in women and inability to ejaculate in men are also common. Younger men with localized prostate cancer and normal presurgical sexual function prior to radical prostatectomy treatment are more likely to recover sexual functioning within 1 year, but substantial numbers of survivors of prostate cancer report erectile dysfunction (Schover et al., 2002). Female breast cancer patients and patients with gynecological cancer commonly experience vaginal dryness and low libido during and following treatment. Ovarian and other gynecologic cancers of the cervix, vagina, vulva, or uterus are all associated with sexual dysfunction (Maiorino et al., 2016). Cancers of the male reproductive system, such as testicular cancer, also are associated with sexual difficulties. Localized testicular cancer has a very high (95%) survival rate and usually occurs in men between the ages of 20 and 39; the risk for lasting sexual side effects is high. Risk factors for sexual dysfunction in people with colon cancer are location of the cancer, type of surgery, radiation therapy, presence of a stoma, and older age (Traa, De Vries, Roukema, & Den Oudsten, 2012).

Surgery, radiation therapy, and some types of chemotherapy substantially influence interest in or ability to enjoy sexual intercourse. Androgen deprivation therapy for metastatic prostate cancer is associated with lower testosterone levels, reduced libido, and decreases in the size and length of the penis (Kim, 2011). Aromatase inhibitors used to treat breast cancer can cause symptoms such as vaginal dryness and decreased desire.

Health care professionals often do not feel comfortable discussing sexual concerns with patients. Many disciplines assume that it falls under another provider's purview or feel that they lack the necessary time and/or communication skills. Surprisingly, some physicians feel it is inappropriate to introduce sexual functioning unless the patient brings up the topic. Members of the American Radiology Society were surveyed ($N = 799$) and results revealed that 64% to 78% of providers never or rarely discuss sexual functioning with patients (Koontz et al., 2012). Female providers and those with more experience are more likely to ask patients about sexual functioning. Importantly, provider perception of the importance of sexual function to their patient appears to influence the frequency of discussion, and 43% of providers indicate that they feel more training in discussing sexual concerns would be helpful. Ideally, sexual functioning should be assessed before, during, and after cancer treatment. Patients report that they would like to know whether sexual functioning is likely to be affected by treatment, to understand the cause of dysfunction and the potential duration of sexual side effects, to have specific examples of dysfunction, and to know when it is safe to resume sexual intercourse (Stead, Brown, Fallowfield, & Selby, 2003).

Exploration of emotional responses to sexual dysfunction is even more complex than discussion of the direct sexual side effects of treatment. Grief and feelings of loss are appropriate reactions to the loss of normal bodily functions such as erection upon awakening, spontaneous erection, and physical sensation. This topic is sensitive and emotionally laden. Many medical treatments are experienced as traumatizing by a proportion of patients. Mastectomy is an example of a potentially traumatic surgery that leaves some individuals unwilling to be touched or seen by their partner. Women who have undergone mastectomy frequently experience painful lymphedema following surgery, and these types of symptoms are associated with higher risk for sexual problems. Men and women frequently report feelings of embarrassment related to inability to achieve an erection or dyspareunia.

Cognitive restructuring can be used to change underlying beliefs that sexual functioning is completely dependent upon ability to achieve erection or have intercourse. Guided imagery, sexual fantasy, and relaxation techniques are effective in reducing anxiety and increasing sexual enjoyment. Psychoeducation about self-stimulation helps to normalize fears and reduce feelings of embarrassment. Facilitation of open discussion of sexual exploration, massage, and nonsexual touch between partners helps to maintain a sense of both emotional and sexual connection.

YOUNG ADULTS

Young adults with cancer have the challenging predicament of concern about cancer recurrence, fear of a foreshortened lifespan, and feelings of isolation. Young adults who are not in relationships but want to have a partner in the future face the difficult challenge of deciding what to disclose about their cancer history when dating. Some dating partners are unable or unwilling to go forward in a relationship because they feel overwhelmed, ill equipped, or fearful about the impact of cancer on their future. This in turn can create deep feelings of rejection, grief, and anger about yet another loss to cancer. The impact of losing a valued relationship with a potential life partner because of cancer history may create loss of trust and damage to self-esteem. Discussions of fertility are not typically advisable in the early stages of a dating relationship, and some patients report feeling like there is never a good time or way to broach the subject. Partners of young adults diagnosed with cancer often feel considerable guilt if they want to end the relationship, regardless of the reason. Psychotherapy for each of the individuals and the couple can help them gain some much-needed perspective at a crucial time.

FERTILITY PRESERVATION

Most cancers occur later in life, but about 5% of all cancer cases occur between the ages of 15 and 39 years (American Cancer Society, 2016). Many types of cancer treatments present high risk for infertility for young adults. When survival is at stake, it is easy to overlook or minimize discussion of infertility. Fertility preservation efforts must take place before treatment, but the time window to comprehend the implications of a cancer diagnosis, obtain information about the impact on fertility, and take action is narrow. Fertility preservation guidelines in oncology have existed in the United States for little more than a decade (Loren et al., 2013).

The most effective methods of preserving fertility are sperm and embryo banking, although a variety of technological advances have created other good options as well. Embryo banking in turn often creates the extremely complicated challenges of financing fertility treatment and choosing a gestational carrier. Even after a successful implantation, miscarriage may occur, giving rise to more feelings of loss in a person who has already undergone the extraordinary burden of coping with potentially life-threatening illness. Women of reproductive age who are undergoing fertility treatment after cancer benefit from psychological intervention to help with decision making. Psychological treatment can facilitate exploration of the patient's view on the pros and cons of the available fertility treatment options. The decision can be influenced by medical factors, as well as relationship status and spiritual beliefs. Many people find that it is easier to discuss the impact of the possible decision on their future quality of life, health, financial well-being and relational satisfaction with the therapist as a neutral third party. Ethical considerations, such as how long to store the sperm, eggs, or embryo, and the conditions (if any) in which these can be used in the future require high levels of decision-making ability at a time when emotional resources are often depleted.

Whether to use donations from a third party (sperm, embryos) is a decision that can be made after treatment for cancer is completed. Cancer survivors who have a donor or gestational carrier who is known (e.g., a friend, relative) sometimes report persistent feelings of guilt or ambivalence. Decisions about whether to use donor sperm, to adopt in the future, or not to have children at all are complex for an adult diagnosed with cancer during their reproductive years. To patients, it can feel very life affirming to focus on having a child following cancer treatment. But for patients, partners, and family members, the usual unspoken fear is that the cancer may recur. Women who were already planning or have started a family often feel a need to have a child as quickly as possible for a variety of reasons. Those with children may want to have the next child as close in age as possible. Frequently, the anticipation of difficulties in implanting an embryo drives the decision to move forward quickly. Often, people do not have enough time to process the psychological impact of having had cancer before embarking on the stressful path to parenthood.

BODY IMAGE

Cancer and its treatment affect body image, both directly and indirectly. Surgeries such as mastectomy have been well studied, and it is normal that such a radical surgery affects body image to some degree in the short term, even in the most resilient people. Although body image has been most studied in women with mastectomy, any cancer treatment that results in permanent or temporary disfigurement can leave a person uncomfortable with having bandage dressings changed, being touched, or looking at their own scars. Cancer survivors frequently express concern about their desirability to a partner. Some cancer survivors express reluctance to undress in front of a partner. Some may wonder whether others can tell they were treated for cancer. Women face challenges in finding appropriate, comfortable clothing such as swimwear and bras following mastectomy, especially if they face financial stress.

Symptoms such as fatigue may give rise to feeling old, and this too can make a person feel less attractive. Weight gain due to chemotherapy is associated with substantial negative feelings. The induction of a menopausal state with its concomitant symptoms such as hot flashes is psychologically challenging for premenopausal women. The technology of prosthetics has made dramatic strides, but prosthetic devices can be extremely difficult for some people to accept. The psychological impact of prosthetics involving a limb or facial part is very different from the impact of reconstructive breast surgery. Psychological support for decision making related to prosthetics is often lacking. People with gastrointestinal cancer who need a stoma experience profound impact on their sense of bodily integrity. Ports are usually placed on the upper chest, and this too can create negative feelings and challenges if the person wants to wear clothes that hide the port in warm weather. Some ports are placed in areas that are easily seen, such as the head (for some patients with brain tumor), causing the patient to feel self-conscious in public. It is normal to have some level of negative feeling about the effect of cancer on feelings of attractiveness and body integrity. Although distress is a common reaction to cancer treatment and is usually transient, psychological treatment can help to decrease its intensity and duration.

Exploration of body image concerns requires a good understanding of the patient's feelings about the body prior to treatment. Patients often express the feeling that their concerns are unwarranted—"I feel silly complaining about this [body image concern] when I see so many other people in the waiting room fighting for their life" is an often-heard sentiment.

HAIR LOSS

Some people fear hair loss associated with some chemotherapeutic agents even more than cancer itself, whereas others do not feel that hair loss is a significant burden. Frequently, patients who are losing their hair during cancer treatment cut it shorter or shave it, perhaps to gain some measure of control. Some patients struggle with hair loss to such a degree that as their hair becomes sparse, they are unwilling to go out in public any more than necessary. The continuum of hair loss can range from total (including eyebrows and eyelashes) to mild hair thinning. Hair is a cultural marker of desirability, attractiveness, and health, so it is not surprising that hair loss has significant psychological consequences.

For some, hair loss is an outward indicator of illness and can trigger feelings of vulnerability. A mental health professional can help patients verbalize their fears. Cognitive behavioral therapy that focuses on anticipated questions or potentially uncomfortable situations and rehearsal of coping strategies increases confidence in social situations. In particular, parents of younger children often state that they fear that their children will be more worried about them because of hair loss. Therapists can help normalize patients' feelings about hair loss and help them weigh the pros and cons of decisions, such as whether to wear a wig. Connection with another cancer survivor who has also undergone hair loss also offers valuable support.

Maintaining a positive body image during and after cancer treatment can be challenging. A cognitive approach to therapy focuses on identifying and challenging automatic negative thoughts (e.g., "Everyone thinks I'm dying"). Self-monitoring by keeping a journal to record thoughts and emotions associated with body image is useful. Assigning homework (e.g., making a list of positive things the person likes about themselves, keeping a gratitude journal) can play a role in shifting body image perceptions to a more benign or neutral view.

SUMMARY

Oncologists and other health care providers do not have sufficient time to have more nuanced discussions of sexual side effects or body image. Therefore, assessment of sexual concerns and possible worries about physical appearance is critical at the earliest stages of mental health treatment. Because people are often reticent to bring up their concerns to a provider, they may endure long-term suffering from problems that might have been treatable.

8

Impact of Cancer Diagnosis and Treatment on the Family, and the Role of Social Support

Strong, supportive relationships make a cancer diagnosis easier to bear. People who have few social ties or who have distressed relationships face more difficulty with both the emotional and logistical issues involved with treatment. Cancer also takes a tremendous toll on loved ones, and spouses have rates of anxiety that are similar to patients themselves (Mitchell, Ferguson, Gill, Paul, & Symonds, 2013). Because family members play a critical role in influencing a patient's treatment, their involvement in care is paramount. The role of the caregiver is taxing, and resources to address the intense psychological demands of supporting a loved one with a serious health problem are inadequate. In clinical settings, most psychosocial outpatient resources are designed to meet the needs of patients rather than family members. Ideally, holistic psychosocial oncology care should assess the needs of both the person living with cancer and their immediate family (partners and spouses,

http://dx.doi.org/10.1037/0000054-009
Psychological Treatment of Patients With Cancer, by E. A. Dornelas
Copyright © 2018 by the American Psychological Association. All rights reserved.

adult children in a caretaking role, younger children). This type of assessment has been described in medical family therapy textbooks (McDaniel, Doherty, & Hepworth, 2014).

CAREGIVER BURDEN

The vast majority of research related to family members of people diagnosed with cancer has focused on spouses/partners, and a great proportion of that scientific work has been devoted to describing the problem of caregiver burden. By definition, a caregiver may provide tangible support, such as financial assistance or transportation, as well as emotional, physical, and spiritual support. Caregivers often become the patient's advocate, schedule appointments, and educate themselves about diagnoses and treatments. Caregivers may overextend themselves if they simultaneously cope with increased child care burden and/or becoming the primary wage earner. Rates of anxiety and depression in caregivers range from 10% to 50% (Mitchell et al., 2013). Risk and resiliency factors for caregiver burden are described in Table 8.1. Cancer diagnoses associated with greater functional impairment (e.g., brain tumors) place a tremendous strain on caregivers, who may need to completely restructure their lives temporarily

Table 8.1
Risk and Resiliency Factors for Caregiver Burden

Risk factors	Resiliency factors
Caring for homebound spouse	Strong network of support
Low socioeconomic status	Greater access to financial resources
Coping with own health problems	Flexible working conditions
Progression of disease	Engagement in social activities
Relational distress	Help with other care giving responsibilities
Inability to accept caregiving role	(e.g., child care, elder care)
Health-risk behaviors (e.g., alcohol abuse)	Healthy lifestyle/exercise
Avoidant coping	Problem-solving orientation

or permanently to adjust to the demands of the treatment and the disease. The length of time to be spent caregiving is unknown at the outset, but the role and its tasks can extend for years.

COUPLES AND CANCER

The majority of cancer caregivers are over the age of 65 and caring for spouses of about the same age (Girgis et al., 2013). Women are more likely to be in caregiving roles, and fatigue is the most often cited health impact of taking care of a partner with cancer (Clark et al., 2014). The physical health impact of caregiving is not trivial. In-home caregiving to a disabled spouse is associated with higher risk for stroke, with the highest associations seen for men and particularly African American men (Haley, Roth, Howard, & Safford, 2010).

Assessment of the partner/spouse as well as the person diagnosed with cancer includes exploration of their understanding about the diagnosis/ prognosis, available resources for support, and ability for self-care. A lifespan developmental approach can inform assessment, as the needs of each couple dyad vary widely. People with cancer may have long-term, committed relationships or marriages that are healthy or distressed. Even in the healthiest of relationships, coping with a partner's cancer diagnosis is difficult. The spouse without cancer who has their own health problems may feel stressed about the loss of a supportive partner or worried about their financial future. Couples with preexisting marital stress face unique difficulties with increased resentment, anger, regret, or guilt that in turn can complicate the course of illness. Schnarch (1997) said that a reality of long-term marriage is that one partner winds up burying the other. Although this is inevitable, rarely does any individual think through what this might be like until they face such a situation. Cancer can be "the elephant in the room" that is never discussed. An anecdotal example of a common communication difficulty is a spouse who longs for verbal expressions of appreciation while the person with cancer is often simply too sick to engage in abstract thought or may have never been an emotionally expressive individual. Avoidant communication patterns are associated with higher distress levels (Manne et al., 2006). Thus, although cancer brings some couples closer together, it can also be very isolating for both parties. Badr, Gupta, Sikora, and Posner (2014) examined patient–partner dyads and found that increased distress in one partner is associated with increased distress in the other. They hypothesized that the dyad manages distress together as a unit. This line of research implies that supportive interventions with a dyadic approach can be effective at reducing distress for both patient and partner (Badr et al., 2014).

Problem-solving therapy (PST) is a structured approach that has been shown to benefit partners of people with cancer (Meyers et al., 2011). PST teaches generalizable problem solving skills. Couples coping with cancer face logistical and emotionally complex situations, and PST increases confidence in ability to successfully navigate those challenges.

Nontraditional couples may benefit from supportive interventions for the dyad. This topic is discussed in more detail later in the section on the impact of cancer on lesbian, gay, bisexual, and transgender (LGBT) couples. However, nontraditional couples include anyone who is cohabitating, in a committed relationship but not cohabitating, and close friends who function as each other's primary support. In addition to dealing with cancer, these couples can face stressors related to legal and financial matters, family estrangement or discord, lack of emotional or social support, and lack of recognition by the medical community for their role in their partner's life (e.g., policies such as hospital visiting hours that are open only to "family").

IMPACT OF CANCER ON YOUNG FAMILIES

It is heartrending to work with a parent who asks for help about how to communicate with their young children about a cancer diagnosis. The age of the child or children should guide this discussion, with more complex information relayed as is appropriate for the developmental level of the child. In general, children are best prepared when they are provided with age-appropriate information about the parent's diagnosis and treatment and how these may influence their daily life and routine. It is easier if both parents have been able to process their own emotions related to the diagnosis. Advice from a mental health professional experienced in psychosocial oncology can help parents find the right words, to prepare what they want to say, and to practice with the emotional tone that they want to convey to their children. Side effects from treatment, such as hair loss, should be discussed. Reactions to such side effects are varied; some adolescents may find it embarrassing that their parent has lost their hair, and some children view hair growing back as a sign that the parent is no longer sick. Fatigue, pain, and nausea are invisible to family members, and it can be very frustrating for the patient, child or children, and/or spouse to explain or understand why the person undergoing treatment appears to look the same but cannot keep up with their normal functional abilities. Most adults equate the word *cancer* with death, so it is not surprising that kids who have a parent with cancer wonder whether their parent will die, and this perception is affected by firsthand knowledge of other people (e.g., grandparents) who have died from cancer. It is challenging to find the right words to communicate openly about a poor prognosis, especially if the patient is having difficulty understanding or accepting it themselves. Parents can be anguished that at the time they most want to provide support for their children, they are fighting a life-threatening illness and may be too exhausted or sick to provide as much emotional support as they might ordinarily.

Optimally, another parental figure can help to bolster the child at this difficult time. However, family configurations and situations vary widely. Single parents may need to help to identify sources of support. Sometimes the parent without cancer copes poorly, denying the diagnosis and engaging in behaviors such as drinking heavily or becoming more distant and unavailable at a time when they are most needed. It is common to encounter parents who seek counseling because they are going through divorces with coparenting agreements and the cancer diagnosis adds an emotionally loaded element to an already stressed family dynamic. Family relationships run the continuum from healthy to extremely damaging. A patient who has pathological character traits can use the cancer diagnosis for secondary gain or to manipulate others (e.g., "If you keep stressing me, it will be your fault if my cancer comes back"). Patients with marital distress may blame their ex-spouse or spouse as a factor in the development of their cancer. A motivational interviewing approach to this common dynamic involves not confronting this perception head on, but instead eliciting from the patient their own motivation to refocus their energy on more constructive ways of thinking.

Emotionally charged family dynamics combined with life-threatening illness have a way of reverberating through the health care system. Providers can become entangled in these complex dynamics, generating multiple referrals to the mental health provider from more than one source (e.g., nurse, physician, patient navigator). These situations can be extremely time consuming and are usually beyond the scope of an acute care outpatient or inpatient psychosocial oncology setting. It is more efficient to provide the family recommendations for obtaining care in their community, rather than trying to intervene directly. It is ideal to help parents to find community mental health providers for their children and/or spouses who can then be available as an additional source of support. A community mental health provider can help their client to process the emotional aspects of living with a person who is undergoing cancer treatment. If the patient has a poor prognosis, that therapist can remain available to help the person cope with their grief and loss. In cases where the therapist works primarily with the family rather than the patient themselves, it can be important that the therapist have an opportunity to meet the patient with cancer.

IMPACT OF CANCER ON LESBIAN, GAY, BISEXUAL, AND TRANSGENDER COUPLES

A mental health professional working with patients who have cancer will encounter LGBT patients. Presumably the proportion of patients with cancer who are LGBT is similar to that of the general population. However, the proportion of people who identify as LGBT varies widely according to age and region of the country. In cities where acceptance is high, greater numbers of people self-identify as LGBT. In most cases, being LGBT has little to no effect on adjustment to cancer. However, partners of those with a cancer diagnosis who have conflicted relationships with one or both parents, or adult children, or who is not openly gay, can experience extreme distress in coping with their loved one's illness. Conflict can be played out in determining who makes important decisions about the patient's care, if they are unable to speak for themselves. It is difficult if the life partner is neither recognized as such nor given the same familial support that a heterosexual spouse would expect to experience. Education of the patient and his or her partner in the early stages of illness about advanced directives and efforts to speak openly and clearly with other key family members can help to defuse this type of potentially volatile situation. Older gay couples are less likely to have adult children; thus, the partner may have an even greater caregiver burden. Few caregiver support groups are available, and those that exist are typically oriented to the needs of heterosexual couples. The needs of LGBT couples coping with cancer often go unrecognized. The LGBT community in the United States faces significant prejudice, and these biases can be enacted overtly or covertly by health care professionals in behaviors toward the patient and/or their life partner. Recognizing that an LGBT family member of a cancer patient may have unique psychosocial stressors and helping the person to develop strategies to address those needs is an extremely important and under-studied aspect of cancer care.

IMPACT OF CANCER ON PEOPLE WITH LOW SOCIAL SUPPORT

People with few social ties or very distressed relationships may perceive themselves as being alone in facing cancer. Some individuals have no social support because they have poor psychological functioning. Relationships developed in the context of health care treatment can become a substitute for family. Some patients reenact their family dynamics with their physicians, nurses, or office staff, for example, rebelling against authority by not complying with medical recommendations or by becoming extremely demanding or dependent. To the extent that experienced health care providers sense when this is occurring, they usually become adept at not getting embroiled in the patient's complicated dynamics. Most physicians and nurses are not familiar with psychodynamic terms such as *transference*, *countertransference*, *projection*, and *projective identification*. But life-threatening illness places a person in a very dependent role with their provider, and psychodynamic terminology is sometimes relevant in understanding how the patient is relating to their medical provider.

CASE EXAMPLE

Alicia, an impoverished single mother with major mental illness, utilized more of the cancer center resources than dozens of other patients combined. She needed assistance from the navigator to find transportation to appointments and case management to help her with housing and child care. She missed appointments, fought with the office scheduling staff, and rapidly shifted between gratitude and hostility toward her oncologist. She had no family involved in her life, other than her dependent children. Although family members lived in the immediate vicinity, Alicia seemed to have burned all her bridges.

In this particular example, multidisciplinary intervention focused on support involved a social worker, financial counselor, and oncology nurse navigator, as well as a community mental health provider and case management from child protective services. Critical intervention also focused on providing the treating physician with a framework to understand the patient's anger and to help the provider find ways to avoid engaging while remaining committed to care.

The behavior described in the above example is overwhelming for health care providers. Interpersonally challenging patients are handed off from one provider to another, and delivery of care may not feel particularly rewarding. Ideally, recognizing the dynamics early and developing a team approach to treatment will ameliorate the challenges involved in working with patients who have extremely complex medical, social, and psychological needs.

SOCIOCULTURAL ASPECTS OF WORKING WITH FAMILIES AFFECTED BY CANCER

People of different cultures have tremendously diverse views of cancer, oncology treatment, and dying. Practical issues, such as language barriers, draw adult children into a parent's care more than might ordinarily be expected. Spiritual beliefs (e.g., whether cancer is "God's will") influence a patient's receptiveness to treatment. Also, patients can experience perceived or real stigma from their family. This is especially true for certain cancer diagnoses, such as lung cancer, some gynecological and gastrointestinal cancers, and cancers associated with HIV (e.g., Kaposi's sarcoma). No therapist could have experience with all the potential permutations of how sociocultural factors might influence oncology care. Careful assessment of the patient's background and beliefs is informative as to whether sociocultural factors may play a key role in the family's ability to cope effectively with the cancer diagnosis.

Many patients and/or their family members are inherently distrustful of modern medicine and hence are opposed to chemotherapy, radiation therapy, and/or surgery. This precipitates distress when the patient and family disagree, or when family members themselves disagree, about how to proceed with treatment. In some cases, this distrust may be based on personal knowledge, experience with failures of the health care system, or spiritual beliefs. Sometimes a family's distrust of cancer treatment is an entirely rational and well-thought-out, but in many cases the distrust may not be logical, so it is helpful if the therapist is able to understand the underlying beliefs and thought processes.

IMPACT OF DISEASE PROGRESSION ON SOCIAL SUPPORT

People with metastatic disease that has progressed may have diminishing levels of familial support just at the time that they need it most. If progression occurs many years after the initial diagnosis, the family may underestimate the patient's support needs or be facing their own issues of aging or poor health. The family support needs of patients with advanced cancer are often very different from their needs at the initial diagnosis. Partners, parents, and children experience the initial impact of the patient's first course of illness and treatment as traumatizing, but they can become desensitized or disengaged from the patient as the illness recurs or progresses. It is particularly sad when loved ones draw away from patients who have limited time and a poor prognosis. By assessing support needs and educating family members about the illness and its influence on the family, clinicians can strengthen support for people with advanced metastatic disease.

PSYCHOLOGICAL INTERVENTIONS FOR FAMILIES AFFECTED BY CANCER

A 2010 review of 29 randomized controlled trials of interventions for caregivers offers support for the positive impact of psychological intervention on patients and family members (Northouse, Katapodi, Song, Zhang, & Mood, 2010). Educational interventions, skills training (e.g., coping skills training, communication), and counseling interventions in Northouse et al.'s (2010) meta-analysis included improved marital relationships, self-efficacy, coping ability, and physical functioning, as well as decreased anxiety. From a clinical perspective, the evidence indicates that approaches that focus on promotion of active, problem-solving coping, and decreasing use of avoidant coping strategies have positive outcomes for family members and caregivers.

Stage of illness greatly affects the feasibility of psychological intervention. A review of 23 couples-based interventions indicated that interventions at earlier stages of illness are more effective in reducing anxiety and improving quality of life than interventions delivered at later stages (Regan et al., 2012). Interventions timed at later stages of diagnosis are more likely to positively influence the patient's illness appraisal and feelings of hopelessness, as well as the partner's confidence in their caregiving ability. A study of women with early-stage breast cancer found that couples with high levels of distress and those in which the partner is perceived to be unsupportive appear to derive the greatest degree of benefit from intervention (Manne, Ostroff, Winkel, Grana, & Fox, 2005).

Historically, behavioral interventions are usually delivered face-to-face, but caregivers, life partners, family members, and patients often have little availability or free time. Delivery of psychological intervention can take place individually, in group format with patient and the family members, or with the family member or members alone. Intervention can be conducted in person, by telephone, via the Internet, or some combination thereof. More research examining the delivery of telephone, web-based, and other telehealth counseling interventions is needed because these potentially offer greater logistical flexibility and greater perceived anonymity, and may be more cost-effective.

Finally, most research on the impact of cancer on couples, families, and caregivers has been conducted with White, well-educated men and women with prostate or breast cancer. The need is pressing to examine the family support needs of racial and ethnic minority patients and of LGBT patients, as well as to test psychological interventions to address those needs.

9

Posttreatment Psychological Sequelae

Advances in oncology treatment have dramatically increased long-term cancer survival rates. Many cancer treatments are curative, leaving survivors with no evidence of disease or long periods of time in remission. But the possibility of recurrence remains for all cancer survivors. From a medical perspective, cancer follow-up is similar to managing a chronic disease in terms of the need for ongoing pharmacological treatment, surveillance, and secondary prevention through changing health behaviors. More than 15.5 million cancer survivors live in the United States, a number that is expected to grow to 20 million by 2026 (American Cancer Society, 2016); thus, many people who have been treated for cancer are expected to be long-term survivors. Considerable psychological adjustment is necessary to assimilate the meaning of a cancer diagnosis and to adapt to a "new normal" life as a survivor.

http://dx.doi.org/10.1037/0000054-010
Psychological Treatment of Patients With Cancer, by E. A. Dornelas
Copyright © 2018 by the American Psychological Association. All rights reserved.

SURVIVORSHIP

Cancer survivorship refers to the movement to recognize and study the long-term psychological and physical effects of cancer treatment. The Commission on Cancer implemented a 2015 standard to ensure that all patients receive a survivorship care plan, which includes two primary components: (a) a treatment summary and (b) a follow-up care plan that includes information such as potential late side effects and written recommendations that address posttreatment surveillance and follow-up care. Quality Oncology Practice Initiative standards from the American Society of Clinical Oncology also include guidelines related to cancer survivorship. Cancer survivorship programs aim to help patients to feel more knowledgeable and confident about their health following treatment. The health care system in the United States is fragmented compared with countries such as Denmark (Dalton, Mellemkjaer, Olsen, Mortensen, & Johansen, 2002), and few American health networks have optimally integrated electronic medical records. Patients typically complete treatment without a full understanding of the results of their surgery, types of chemotherapies used, and/or details about their radiation treatment. In the initial upheaval after diagnosis, people are most anxious to get started with life-saving treatment, and it is understandable that patients would pay less attention to the remote threat of potential long-term side effects of cancer treatment. For example, many types of chemotherapy and radiation therapy are associated with risk for cardiac disease, particularly congestive heart failure. Yet, relatively few patients understand this risk or know enough about symptoms of cardiomyopathy to recognize early warning signs of heart failure. A diagnosis of cancer increases the risk for future cancers, even in people with curable disease. Long-term survivors with recurrence who were treated in the pre-Internet age have difficulty in obtaining the original images or details of their treatment. It is common that patients do not understand the role each specialty physician (e.g., medical oncologist, surgeon, radiation oncologist) played in their care or even have the names of their providers. A treatment summary provides the details of the patient's cancer, their treatment, and the contact information for the professionals involved in their care. Health care systems increasingly use a portal to make such information more easily accessible to the patient. As the person's treatment evolves, the survivorship care plan and treatment summary become "living documents" that are updated in real time. This information is invaluable to the patient, as well as to the physician who eventually assumes responsibility for long-term surveillance. Included in the many models for survivorship care are ones in which the patient may be followed by their medical oncologist, by a physician assistant or an advanced practice nurse in the oncologist's practice, in a survivorship care clinic, or by their primary care physician (PCP). The survivorship care plan is particularly intended to inform the PCP about the patient's specific follow-up needs.

Commonly, patients become confused about whether their long-term follow-up should be managed by their medical oncologist, surgeon, or PCP. From a psychological perspective, the medical oncologist is often viewed as the person who has literally saved their life, and so it is understandable that patients are reluctant to entrust their long-term surveillance to another provider. Medical oncologists who do not transition patients in long-term surveillance to a different provider will be buried under the load of patient care. Education is needed for PCPs about their role in follow up of people treated for cancer and for improved cross communication between primary care and oncology. A survivorship visit is ideally timed at the end of treatment. The visit involves an assessment of the person's psychological status, support needs, sexual functioning, physical functioning, and health-risk behaviors. The assessment identifies areas of concern and should include patient-reported outcomes and a medical exam. The goal of a survivorship care plan is to provide education that will promote healthy behaviors, improve quality of life, and ensure awareness of the need to monitor for late side effects. A survivorship care plan also provides the patient with a connection to appropriate resources (e.g., psychological treatment, nutritionist).

FEAR OF RECURRENCE AND DISEASE PROGRESSION

Most people with early- and late-stage cancer fear the disease's recurrence or progression. For some people, despite assurance of excellent prognosis, this fear persists for many years. The problem is important because fear of recurrence is associated with poor quality of life (Sarkar et al., 2014).

Anxiety about an uncertain future is understandable, but disproportionate worry about recurrence should be assessed further and (if necessary) treated. People who are younger, have greater levels of distress, or have more symptoms are at highest risk for disproportionate fear of recurrence (Crist & Grunfeld, 2013). Many cancer survivors become anxious when they experience common symptoms, such as headache, backache, or other symptoms, and find it difficult to gauge when it is the appropriate time to contact their physician. Reviewing the onset, duration, and reason for the worry, as well as the context of other potential stressors in the person's life, is important. People may fail to see other patterns in their lives that give rise to stress (e.g., marital discord), which can make them more vulnerable to interpret bodily symptoms or sensations as evidence of recurrence or disease progression. For example, many people with stable metastatic disease report that common headaches cause worry that cancer has metastasized to the brain. Excessive stress in other aspects of life increases this likelihood. Online social networks for people with cancer can provide support. But interaction with a member who experiences recurrence or disease progression can trigger worry in other people in the group. A mental health provider can help the cancer survivor to weigh the pros and cons of online education and support and can help to objectively evaluate whether the survivor is deriving enough benefit and can tolerate hearing information about other members that may hit too close to home. Fear of recurrence that is manifested by a high degree of worry about somatic symptoms should respond to a cognitive approach (Lebel et al., 2014; Simard et al., 2013) that includes an understanding of the basic cognitive behavioral therapy (CBT) model; being able to discriminate between appropriate concern versus catastrophic thinking; and keeping a journal to write down symptoms as they occur, noting the onset, duration, and other potential stressors. Psychotherapy is helpful in gaining the perspective that the prospect of cancer recurrence is understandably frightening, but excessive focus on somatic symptoms is not likely to result in earlier detection of recurrence and definitely has a negative impact on quality of life.

A different manifestation of fear of recurrence or disease progression involves feeling fatalistic, hopeless, and preoccupied with death (Ozga et al.,

2015). People with a prior history of depression or who tend to score low on the dispositional trait of optimism are more likely to report this cluster of negative thoughts. If untreated or undertreated depression exists, assessment and appropriate treatment should considerably lessen preoccupation with death and hopelessness. If the individual is not depressed but is prone to a negative outlook, is it possible to change this character trait? Mental health professionals know that optimism involves the expectation of positive outcomes. There is a wealth of evidence indicating that optimists cope more effectively with stress in general, are more likely to have good health habits, and have better adjustment to a variety of types of cancers (Geirdal & Dahl, 2008). By keeping expectations low, cancer survivors may be more psychologically prepared to cope with recurrence.

Mental health professionals can also help cancer survivors with fear of recurrence by ascertaining the degree to which they ruminate. Rumination, or the tendency to get "stuck" in a loop of negative thinking, is correlated with many deleterious physiological stress reactions. Like a dog with a bone, the ruminating cancer survivor reviews the negative expectation or thought over and over, unable to let it go. Rumination is conquered in part by learning skills to become engaged in other, more adaptive activities. Shame, guilt, and self-blame are not adaptive and cause a great deal of suffering. Rumination-focused CBT has shown promise for people with depression and aims to identify the maladaptive cognition or emotion and teach skills to shift to more adaptive thinking (Watkins et al., 2011).

People with an optimistic disposition are more likely to exhibit a "fighting spirit" (Hodges & Winstanley, 2012), which is conceptually similar, or possibly related to, the tendency to be persistent in problem-solving efforts and staying engaged in day-to-day activities. Developing skills to notice what is going right by writing down things that were positive each day helps individuals to be more attuned to neutral and positive events, something that comes more naturally for those scoring high on dispositional optimism. Behavioral activation strategies that counter avoidance, withdrawal, and inactivity (Jacobson, Martell, & Dimidjian, 2001) also have merit for people coping with cancer (Hopko, Robertson, & Colman, 2008).

Fear of recurrence or disease progression is a challenging issue for the therapist because of the many logical reasons for such concern. People with advanced cancer who struggle with fear of recurrence need a different approach than those who are disease free. A study testing the effect of CBT and supportive-expressive therapy compared with usual care found that people with advanced disease derive the greatest benefit from psychotherapeutic treatment and that CBT is more cost-effective than nondirective supportive-expressive therapy (Sabariego, Brach, Herschbach, Berg, & Stucki, 2011). The hard fact remains that a history of cancer increases the likelihood of another cancer, even for people with curable disease. When cancer does recur, it is inevitably stressful and demoralizing, and usually triggers memories of prior treatment. This topic is covered in the section that follows.

CANCER RECURRENCE

Cancer recurrence is a powerful emotional experience. People who have had cancer thought to be curable may be bewildered to learn that they have experienced recurrence or developed a new cancer. Those with metastatic disease that has been stable for a period of years are often similarly surprised to learn that their disease has progressed. Cancer recurrence is associated with risk for depression in vulnerable individuals (Step, Kypriotakis, & Rose, 2013). Unlike a first diagnosis of cancer, people may perceive that they have exhausted their support network. Advanced metastatic disease makes it difficult to accomplish things that were previously part of a daily routine (e.g., taking care of children, working, doing household chores). Studies of women with recurrent breast cancer indicate that it is critical to learn how to rethink priorities to reengage in important goals. For example, Low and Stanton (2015) found that 78% of women with metastatic breast cancer indicated that they gave up a goal that was very important to them because of the disease. Goals such as completing a degree, traveling to another country, or being involved in a sport can become unachievable when cancer recurs. Half of all women in Low and Stanton's sample curtailed at least one activity, and 39% had clinically significant symptoms using the Center for Epidemiologic Studies Depression Scale measure cutoff of greater than or equal to 16. The researchers hypothesized that the more activity is disrupted, the less a woman would feel positive affect. Psychological treatment that focuses on problem solving, regaining a sense of control, setting new goals for the future, and promoting a fighting spirit are effective at improving positive affect in people with metastatic disease. Supportive-expressive therapy delivered over the course of a year is effective in reducing symptoms of depression, feelings of hopelessness/ helplessness, and trauma symptoms, and improving social support in women with metastatic breast cancer (Kissane et al., 2007). Supportive-expressive therapy is a 12-week group intervention with 90-minute sessions that has been widely used with cancer populations (Classen et al., 2008). Supportive-expressive group therapy for oncology patients focuses on developing a support network within the group and improving relationships with family and medical caregivers.

Anger is an understudied topic in psychosocial oncology but is a commonly expressed emotion in clinical practice in both individual and group therapy settings. Anger experienced following the end of treatment is understandable, particularly in cases where a diagnosis was missed, the patient had a negative experience with the health care system, or cancer has progressed or recurred. Anger may be directed toward anyone, but most often caregivers, medical practitioners, and coworkers bear its brunt. Anger is an adaptive emotion in that it mobilizes the individual to appropriately assert their needs, but persistent irritable mood is problematic and may be ego syntonic. Gentle education about how to recognize anger is necessary before an individual can begin to address the problem. Eliciting the array of ways in which anger may be manifested—including but not limited to vocal tone and volume, facial expressions, resentful thoughts, physiological arousal, sarcasm, explosiveness, aggressive behavior/combativeness, and withdrawal—is an important precursor to engaging a person into efforts to address the problem. Convincing evidence indicates that hostility is predictive of mortality in healthy populations and recurrence of heart disease (Smith, Glazer, Ruiz, & Gallo, 2004). In contrast, the link between hostility and cancer is not well established. Maladaptive anger is an emotionally dysregulated state, but it is overregulation of anger (greater anger control and suppression of anger) that is correlated with mortality risk in the oncology population (Chapman, Fiscella, Kawachi, Duberstein, & Muennig, 2013). Emotional suppression of anger is associated with shorter survival times in women with breast cancer (Lehto, Ojanen, Dyba, Aromaa, & Kellokumpu-Lehtinen, 2007; Reynolds et al., 2000) and with lower levels of natural killer cell cytotoxicity in men with localized prostate cancer (Penedo et al., 2006). Chronic anger suppression takes a toll on the body. When expressed in a maladaptive way, anger can trigger behaviors that are later a source of regret and shame.

Anger is most likely to be experienced in the context of human relationships (e.g., patient–caregiver, doctor–patient, parent–child), and cancer puts tremendous strain on relational ties. The context of cancer is challenging. The person who chronically suppresses healthy, appropriate anger believes that it is important to control their feelings, and in the context of postcancer treatment, may feel guilty about the anger. The mental health professional can help by validating anger as a healthy emotional response and identifying constructive ways to express the feeling or assert oneself when needed. It is important to challenge the belief that suppressing anger makes the individual more evolved or places them on higher moral ground. The context of cancer provides a window of opportunity for change. Following treatment, people with the habit of expressing their anger in maladaptive manner sometimes note that cancer places things into perspective and they do not feel as reactive to triggers. Conversely, those who chronically suppress anger may find that following treatment, they see themselves as having a right to their emotions and feel more comfortable with self-assertion.

Negative emotions, particularly depression, can play a greater role in the progression of some types of cancers, such as hormonal cancers (prostate and endometrial) and immune-mediated cancers (e.g., lymphomas; Costanzo, Sood, & Lutgendorf, 2011). Patients who undergo hematopoietic stem cell transplantation are at increased risk for depressive symptoms, which are in turn associated with poorer recovery of immune functioning and shorter survival times (Steel, Geller, Gamblin, Olek, & Carr, 2007). However, the knowledge that negative emotion may play a role in cancer progression can, paradoxically, induce its own form of stress, as the following case example illustrates.

CASE EXAMPLE

Joe was a 60-year-old executive in otherwise good health, diagnosed with an aggressive form of lymphoma. He underwent stem cell transplant and was referred for psychological treatment by his medical oncologist. He presented with severe clinical depression, which responded to CBT and a medication regimen that included both an antidepressant and a stimulant. He described his lifestyle before diagnosis as very stressful and was on long-term partial disability. He expressed the fear that although he had completed treatment, return to full-time work would unduly tax his immune system and could trigger recurrence. CBT-oriented treatment focused on identifying Joe's black-and-white thinking and helping him to proactively find other ways to think about and cope with his anticipated stressors.

FINDING BENEFITS

A growing literature shows that at least half of patients with cancer report some benefit as a result of cancer (Antoni et al., 2001; Cordova, Cunningham, Carlson, & Andrykowski, 2001). People who see benefit in cancer report that they take more pleasure in their relationships with family and friends, have changed their priorities, feel more appreciative of their life, feel more connected to nature, experience a greater sense of spirituality and purpose, and/or have a greater appreciation for their health. A related line of research theorizes that some people are fundamentally changed as a result of posttraumatic growth (Prati & Pietrantoni, 2009). Posttraumatic growth posits that cancer places the individual in a stressful, potentially life-threatening situation and that some people experience psychological maturation or a higher level of functioning as a result. Posttraumatic growth is thought to fall into one of three domains: feelings or perceptions about the self, feelings toward others, and attitudes about life. The clinical implications of this research are not completely clear. One potential implication of notion of illness as a catalyst for posttraumatic growth is that people have the capacity to develop greater resiliency. The stress of cancer tests the ability to cope effectively in the face of adversity. From a longitudinal perspective, although survivors can often point out benefit and report changes indicative of posttraumatic growth, the evidence that some people truly change and become more resilient as a direct result of posttraumatic growth is limited. Mental health clinicians should focus on exploring an individual's emotional reactions following treatment and help patients with cancer to strengthen their coping skills, but this does not translate into pulling for a patient to find benefit or look for growth in their diagnosis. Validating benefits and growth that patients express on their own can be very helpful, but no evidence indicates that psychotherapists should make active efforts to connect cancer and posttraumatic growth in cancer survivors.

COGNITIVE IMPAIRMENT

Little research has investigated cognitive impairment associated with chemotherapy treatment, colloquially referred to as "chemo-brain" and described in Chapter 3. Correlational studies suggest that up to half of patients undergoing chemotherapy for cancer report cognitive complaints, such as deficits in short-term memory and executive function (Lindner et al., 2014). The degree of cognitive impact varies widely and is influenced by many factors. People with premorbid cognitive impairment and older age are most likely to be vulnerable to chemotherapy-related cognitive impairment (Lindner et al., 2014). Very few people have a baseline cognitive assessment before cancer diagnosis and treatment; thus, it is a challenge to objectively evaluate change in cognitive functioning. People with very high premorbid cognitive functioning who experience impairment may find that their complaints are discounted if they drop from an exceptional to an average level of functioning. Even relatively mild cognitive impairment can be debilitating. Patients who complain of cognitive impairment benefit from tracking their cognitive symptoms to help to pinpoint specific areas of deficit. Patients with brain tumors usually undergo neuropsychological evaluation, but this only takes place after the tumor is already identified and, often, treated. People who feel that their cognitive functioning has markedly declined need work-up and surveillance. Untreated depression and anxiety worsens cognitive functioning. Many types of oral chemotherapy are associated with reports of cognitive decline. Metastasis to the brain is almost always associated with cognitive decline. Psychological interventions can help individuals to develop compensatory strategies and aid in restoring their organization skills, memory, and ability to maintain attention. It is important not to dismiss the complaint of cognitive impairment but to evaluate it in the context of premorbid cognitive functioning, length of time since treatment, and with input from the patient's medical oncologist.

Not uncommonly, it is the patient's spouse, adult child, or other caregiver who reports that their loved one shows decline in cognitive skills, but the problem may be unrecognized by the patient. This is an important and delicate area, particularly if potential endangerment is not recognized by the person with cancer (e.g., driving, forgetting to turn the stove off). Working with both the patient and family member to evaluate whether cognitive skills have been affected by cancer or its treatment and developing an appropriate referral or treatment plan are key aspects of a follow-up care plan.

CHOICE OF WORDS

Many people do not like the term *survivor*. Some people report finding the term offensive, particularly if they do not have curable disease. It is interesting to note that in other areas of medicine, it is not common for people to refer to themselves as survivors, for instance, as cardiac survivors, HIV survivors, or Parkinson's survivors, although they too faced life-threatening diseases with the need for life-long surveillance and treatment. Yet, the field of psychosocial oncology has promoted widespread use of the term *survivor*, and entire conferences are devoted to the topic of cancer survivorship. This is good from the standpoint of bringing greater public awareness to the understudied topic of the posttreatment needs of people with cancer. The term resonates with many people. It is not politic to question whether *survivor* is necessarily the right or best term to describe people who are in long-term stable remission. *Chronic cancer* may be a more acceptable term (Tralongo, Annunziata, Santoro, Tirelli, & Surbone, 2013) and less fraught in the context of psychotherapy. Similarly, not all people are receptive to referring to cancer as a "journey." From the clinical perspective, it is wise to choose words carefully and not to assume that people treated for cancer will view themselves as "survivors," find benefit from their "journey," or have the perspective that cancer has been a catalyst for posttraumatic growth. In general, it is a better approach to carefully listen to the patient's experience, assess posttreatment needs, and refer and/or treat psychological concerns.

10

Existential Themes in Cancer Care

Knowledge of the imminence of one's personal death is isolating, and most people experience feelings of fear, grief, helplessness, and hopelessness at the realization. Kris Karr (2008) referred to death as "the big dirt nap" in her book *Crazy, Sexy Cancer Survivor*. It is unusual to find a cancer self-help book that confronts death head-on. Many psychosocial oncology support resources never address death. Helping patients to express and process their thoughts and emotions about the end of life presents a significant clinical challenge for mental health professionals working in the field of oncology. A diagnosis of cancer precipitates fear of death. Anxiety over recurrence persists for most people, even those with treatable cancers. Yet, when the end of life is imminent, it is tremendously psychologically difficult for most people to recognize. People have high rates of depression and distress at the end of life (Barrera & Spiegel, 2014), perhaps reflecting a failure in the field of oncology to provide recognition of

http://dx.doi.org/10.1037/0000054-011
Psychological Treatment of Patients With Cancer, by E. A. Dornelas

distress and support for the dying. This chapter reviews the literature on evidence-based psychotherapeutic approaches that help people cope with the inevitability of death.

It is natural that as humans we protect ourselves from examining the concept of death too closely. Impermanence is hard to fathom, particularly in Western culture. Therapists working with patients who have cancer need to be comfortable talking about death with them. But this is just as difficult for therapists as it is for any health care professional, especially after working with patients or their families over a long period of time. Mental health professionals are no better than any other humans at grappling with the concept of nonexistence. Death is the topic that is easier to put off thinking about until some unspecified future time. Working in oncology might be conceptualized as a method of exposure and systematic desensitization therapy that can stimulate maturational growth in this regard. Intentional thinking that life is finite allows people to more fully savor their relationships and things that bring them pleasure. Working with people who have life-threatening illness forces most therapists to confront or at least become more aware of their own denial, fear, and anxiety about death.

Although fear of death is rational and universal, patients with cancer who are already predisposed to anxiety, depression, and trauma are more likely to experience this fear more intensely (Chochinov, 2006). People with somatic disorders become even more sensitized to bodily cues and can experience the confusion of having both symptoms with a medical explanation and symptoms that appear to be psychogenic in nature. Examples of cultural differences in anxiety about death include African Americans reporting higher levels of fear for the body after death and fear of the unknown, compared with Caucasians being more likely to endorse fear of the dying process (Depaola, Griffin, Young, & Neimeyer, 2003). To have good quality of life and gain relief from fear of death, a cognitive approach involves making a conscious, deliberate effort to accept death as a natural end but at the same time to be mindful of being alive in the present. Cancer survivors whose diagnosis forced them to think a great deal about their own death often report that they are living more fully and authentically as a result. This way of living requires a change in cognition from superficial acknowledgement of the inevitability of death to continued awareness but not rumination over mortality. Individual psychotherapy for patients with cancer focused on control of symptoms, relationships, spirituality, and the purpose of life is associated with less anxiety about death and fewer depressive symptoms.

CASE EXAMPLE

Ann had just reached her 50th birthday when she was unexpectedly diagnosed with advanced pancreatic cancer. Her grief was most intense when she talked about her adolescent daughters. She recognized that she would not be likely to see them reach many milestones, such as prom or graduation from high school. Reflecting, she said,

> I don't feel like I need to spend more time or appreciate my children more, because I have always been that kind of mother. I feel good about that. But I worry that they won't have me. I have always been their protector and am more attuned to their needs than my husband.

Therapy with Ann did not focus on her life's purpose or meaning—she already had been living life in a fully intentional manner. She described herself as "uber-mother" and recognized that she was most comfortable caring for others and not familiar with leaning on anyone else. Often, therapy simply offered a space in which Ann could allow herself to let go of a facade of strength and express her authentic emotions, without tempering them for the benefit of her family. She often asked the rhetorical question "Why did this happen? I was the healthiest person I know!" She immediately answered herself, "But why not me, it's just bad luck of the draw." As she worked through her fears that her husband would be unable to care for their children, their relationship became closer. To cope day-to-day, Ann maintained a delicate balance between denial of her illness and belief that she would die from her disease, possibly within months. She noted that it was impossible to know when she should shift from "keeping everything as normal as possible" to talking more openly with her daughters about her illness and acknowledging the "elephant in the room." Similarly, she questioned when she should stop chemotherapy and was concerned that even her oncologist had unrealistic hopes.

End-of-life articles in peer-reviewed publications are rife with unrealistic, idealized views about dying. In truth, many people often continue to deal with complex medical regimens until they die and suffer considerably from symptoms of the cancer, its treatment, or both. Some patients report that it is impossible not to become angry with well-intentioned people who urge them to maintain hope and not to give up. Perhaps the most therapeutic offering from the mental health professional is to remain available to help the person face and cope with their emotions. However, the wish to remain available raises a host of boundary conundrums. It is difficult to know whether and when to visit a patient who is hospitalized and potentially dying if inpatient work is not already part of the therapist's role. In this respect, the frame of the therapy can be more fluid but also difficult to navigate. The feasibility of visiting a hospitalized patient, determining the right time, deciding how long to stay, and grappling with one's role in that context all present major challenges both logistically and therapeutically. Patients and family members can feel deeply abandoned if they expect to be contacted, but are not, by the therapist when the patient is acutely ill or potentially dying. The best method to manage these expectations is to anticipate and discuss the issues ahead of time.

Many people undergoing cancer treatment make friends with other patients they meet in the treatment setting. Some people develop strong bonds and close friendships with a patient who is in a similar situation. Understandably, a person with cancer who loses a close friend to cancer suffers on many levels. Even if the cancer diagnosis and trajectory are different, it is impossible not to be emotionally affected by firsthand experience of death when the circumstances have personal relevance. The mental health professional can help by asking the friends to anticipate and talk about how they might feel. On the one hand, this type of close friendship can be invaluable, but on the other hand, managing emotions about a friend with cancer requires a great deal of self-awareness and ongoing monitoring to ensure that the friendship continues to be mutually beneficial. Potential targets for psychological intervention at the end of life are described in Table 10.1.

Many people with end-stage cancer report that they feel less focused on their own death but are worried about the effect their illness and death

Table 10.1

Potential Psychological Targets for Intervention at End of Life

Common themes	Potential psychological targets
Reduced functional capability	Develop collaborative, achievable goals with priorities of patient in mind
	Identify at least one pleasurable activity each day
Grief and greater awareness of end of life	Prioritize values (e.g., time with family)
	Explore spiritual beliefs
Caregiver burnout	Self-care
	Supportive therapy
	Referral to support group for caregivers
Hopelessness/anxiety	Meaning making and acceptance
	Differentiate realistic concerns from maladaptive worry

will have on their loved ones. It seems unfair that a patient who is terminally ill should have to both manage their own emotions and worry about the feelings of the people they love. In this respect, the psychotherapist can provide support for the very different needs of both the patient and the family member or friend. Common fears include becoming dependent on others for care, bedridden, unconscious, attached to a catheter, and being unable to maintain personal hygiene. Oncology patients with pain or breathlessness express the fear that their pain will be uncontrollable or that they will die gasping for breath. Discussion of these concerns and the wishes of the dying person in the final days of life alleviates anxiety. Unfortunately, hospice care is usually introduced at a later point in the illness trajectory than is optimal (National Hospice and Palliative Care Organization, 2014). Hospice care requires a physician to certify that the person is not expected to live more than 6 months. Active treatment is ceased in hospice care, although palliative care is continued. The patient must sign a statement indicating that they understand that they are entering into hospice care. Palliative care is not synonymous with hospice care. Palliative care provided to give symptom relief and optimize quality of life and is described in more detail in the section that follows.

PALLIATIVE CARE

The American Society of Clinical Oncology has released provisional guide-lines related to palliative care (Ferrell et al., 2016). *Palliative care* is broadly defined, but essential components include assessment and treatment of symptom distress and functional impairment, relationship building between provider and patient/caregiver, education about illness, assessment of coping needs, coordination with other providers, and clarification of treat-ment goals. Palliative care is interdisciplinary, can encompass the inpatient and outpatient settings, and can be provided via face-to-face interaction, referral to other providers, or by telephone. Palliative care should be introduced early, preferably within 8 weeks of diagnosis for people with advanced cancer and can be given in conjunction with active cancer treat-ment. It is effective in improving patient and caregiver quality of life and decreasing symptom distress (Kavalieratos et al., 2016).

The idea of a "good death" in U.S. culture is associated with being pain free, able to maintain control of basic bodily functions, able to talk with family and friends, and able to die in one's sleep without experi-encing a prolonged period of unconsciousness. This concept is not uni-versally shared across cultures. Some cultures associate suffering with atonement. In many cultures where the role of the eldest son is critical, his presence at a parent's death is highly important. Many people do not believe in the use of pain medication, even when dying, and this can cause conflict between family members. An understanding of what a "good death" means to the patient and their loved ones is best achieved when the patient is not imminently dying. Therapists should be aware of their own cultural values and biases about dying before attempting to undertake this work.

The American concept of a good death is not the reality for most people. A 2013 Gallup Poll found that 70% of those surveyed (more than 1,500 adults) effectively supported euthanasia and agreed that "a doctor should be allowed to end the patient's life by some painless means" if the patient and his or her family request it (when worded differently, far fewer people supported it; Saad, 2013). The movement to provide medical aid in dying that began in Oregon is gaining momentum in the United States.

Having the option to exercise the right to die on one's own terms resonates with many people, including physicians. A 2014 survey of 21,000 physicians across a wide range of specialties, in the United States and Europe, was conducted by Medscape (Kane, 2014). More than half (54%) of physicians agreed with the following statement:

> I believe terminal illnesses such as metastatic cancers or degenerative neurological diseases rob a human of his/her dignity. Provided there is no shred of doubt that the disease is incurable and terminal, I would support a patient's decision to end their life, and I would also wish the same option was available in my case should the need arise.

Support decreases if the question is worded as "physician assisted suicide" rather than "allowing a physician to end a patient's life" painlessly, suggesting that the words used to frame the message substantially influences public perception and support of medical aid in dying.

EXISTENTIAL APPROACHES

Existential therapy originates from existential philosophy, a theory positing that each human being has the responsibility to live life authentically and with meaning. Existential work in therapy involves helping people to express their sense of grief and loss about the realistic prospect of dying prematurely before achieving important life goals (e.g., seeing one's child graduate, experiencing the birth of grandchildren). Beliefs about the fairness of life are shattered by terminal illness. A key component of psychological adjustment involves using the diagnosis as a catalyst to shift this belief, accept the diagnosis, and focus on the relationships or activities that have the greatest value. Meaning making is a variant of existential therapy that has been shown to buffer patients with cancer, particularly against hopelessness and depression (Breitbart et al., 2010). Meaning-making therapy is associated with greater improvement in quality of life, decreased symptom burden, and greater spirituality in adults with end-stage cancer when compared with a robust control condition of massage therapy (Greenstein,

2000). In a study with 120 patients, themes such as the legacy of one's life, impermanence, and hope, as well as the personal meaning derived from relationships, love, or career, were explored. This therapeutic approach has also been delivered in group format to patients with advanced cancer. A study conducted by Breitbart et al. (2015) of 253 patients with advanced cancer randomized to meaning-making group therapy or supportive group therapy found that meaning-making group therapy was associated with improvements in quality of life, fewer depressive symptoms, stronger spirituality, less hopelessness, and reduced symptom burden. This therapeutic approach is transdisciplinary and could be delivered by nurses, chaplains, and physicians, in addition to mental health professionals.

DENIAL

Denial is a complex construct. Denial of the imminence of death and denial of fear are two aspects commonly encountered in psychotherapy. Denial can range from overt unwillingness to discuss the possibility of death to minimization or perceptions of having more time to live than is realistic. The majority (85%) of patients with lung cancer have relatively low levels of denial immediately following diagnosis, but as the disease progresses, the level of denial of illness increases (Vos, Putter, van Houwelingen, & de Haes, 2008). Denial protects the individual from being psychologically overwhelmed, and the dying have a right to denial. It has an adaptive aspect. For example, patients with lung cancer with higher levels of denial also report fewer physical symptoms. But the cost and consequences of maladaptive denial are not trivial. The positive correlation between denial and progression of end-stage disease is related to the delay in seeking hospice care at earlier points in the disease trajectory when it could provide the greatest benefit. People are more likely to demonstrate higher levels of denial with their loved ones than with an interviewer (Hinton, 1994). The therapist can ask, "What is your understanding of your disease?" This simple question elicits key information about the person's level of knowledge and acceptance of their disease, their emotional responses and psychological coping strategies. Inconsistencies can be identified and explored with the goal of helping the individual strengthen their ability to face an unbearable topic. Denial or suppression of anxiety is of value when the person has some level of awareness of fear but intentionally chooses not to focus it. But without such self-awareness, anxiety is manifested in many other ways, making it difficult to disentangle. Patients may arrive at the psychologist's door overwhelmed with terror but unable to verbalize their experience. At these moments, simply asking the person who is acutely afraid to put their hand over their heart and to be reminded that they are alive and to focus on their breath can help bring a sense of calm.

SPIRITUALITY AND RELIGION

Nearly all (99%) oncology patients surveyed by the World Health Organization reported that their spirituality or religious belief is an important component of how they cope with cancer (de Camargos, Paiva, Barroso, Carneseca, & Paiva, 2015). Higher religious belief is associated with lower death anxiety in some studies but not others (A. B. Cohen et al., 2005). Many measures have been developed to measure various domains under the umbrella of spirituality and religious belief. These include a sense of transcendence, faith, belief in a higher power, belief in a plan for one's life, belief in life after death, and sense of connection with a higher power or with nature. Religion does not help all people to cope with serious illness. Some report that they question why they developed cancer, feel abandoned by God, or feel that cancer is a punishment from God. Mental health counseling can help people to express and understand the impact that cancer has on their spiritual beliefs. People who struggle with negative religious beliefs (e.g., the concern that cancer is a punishment from God) can be helped with psychological approaches but referral to chaplain services should also be offered.

THERAPY FOR THE DYING

Time limitations create a high level of intensity in working with oncology patients who are dying. It is unlikely that a therapist can successfully adhere strictly to any one theoretical model, and she or he instead must focus on the unique qualities and situation of the individual with whom they are working. The mental health professional can provide support to the patient and/or family. Although knowledge of imminent death is isolating, psychotherapy can reinforce that the person will not be abandoned in their last days. Helping the dying patient to experience their emotions, explore their reactions, and strive for the best possible use of their time makes this type of work uniquely gratifying for many practitioners in the field of psychosocial oncology.

11

Future Directions in Practice and Clinician Self-Care

Cancer care should be designed with mental health treatment completely integrated into the routine delivery of service. Many serious psychosocial problems encountered in oncology are neither assessed nor treated. In part, this represents the low value that the U.S. health care system places on psychological health as measured by the amount of resources apportioned, as well as the seismic changes occurring in the U.S. health care delivery system. The cost of oncology care has increased dramatically in the past decade. The 2013 designation of "breakthrough therapy" by the U.S. Food and Drug Administration expedited the process of approving potentially lifesaving drugs. These changes, in addition to health care reform and strict compliance requirements, have left health care systems scrambling to adapt to the new economics of oncology care. Providers have larger caseloads because of both the increasing numbers of cancer survivors and new cancer cases. Oncology providers spend more time documenting

http://dx.doi.org/10.1037/0000054-012
Psychological Treatment of Patients With Cancer, by E. A. Dornelas

in fragmented electronic medical records, and reimbursement rates continue to shrink, making it unsurprising that the number of oncologists remains constant despite increasing demands to train new providers in the field. The number of physician-owned private practices continues to decrease, in part due to financial pressures, increased compliance requirements, long hours, high patient caseload, and challenges of dealing with drug shortages in the private practice setting. It is not unusual to have less than one social worker for every 1,000 new cancer cases at any given institution. It is rarer to find psychiatrists or psychologists directly employed at cancer centers. This may be due to lack of recognition of the economic payoff of integration of mental health in the oncology specialty practice setting, as well as practical considerations, such as space constraints. The Commission on Cancer (Fineberg, 2008) requires that psychological care be addressed, and this care is typically provided by overburdened social workers. Oncology social workers are expected to provide psychological support to the patient and family, referral services, and guidance on complex financial and health access issues, with few resources. The complex needs of oncology patients are best served when comprehensive mental health services are available within the cancer care treatment setting. Table 11.1 provides descriptions of different psychosocial oncology care modalities.

Effective integration of the psychological and medical care of the cancer patient improves quality of life for patients and caregivers and contributes to better health outcomes. Carlson and Bultz (2003) estimated that at least 20% of patients need to see a psychiatrist to prescribe medication for depression or anxiety and would benefit from individual or group psychological treatment at some point during the cancer experience. An additional 15% need nonpharmacological treatment for distress, and 25% require intervention to address financial and health coverage problems. A Canadian study published in 2001 documented a 23.5% reduction in health care billing costs for women with early-stage breast cancer treated with psychosocial intervention based on cognitive behavioral therapy, compared with usual care (Simpson, Carlson, & Trew, 2001). Medical cost offset of mental health care for patients with cancer has not been well studied, perhaps because the benefits of psychological intervention for this population are relatively

Table 11.1

Factors to Consider in Design of Psychosocial Oncology Services

Psychosocial oncology modalities	Factors to consider
Consultation and referral	Psychological diagnosis
	Needs assessment and treatment recommendations
	Longer sessions of 45 to 90 minutes
Crisis management and triage	Same visit access to onsite mental health provider
	Positive distress screening tied to referral
	Brief sessions of 15 to 30 minutes
Individual therapy	Scheduled outpatient or inpatient visits
	Length of sessions
	Planned goals and length of therapy
	Available to patient and/or family members
Group therapy	Open or closed
	Education, support, and/or psychotherapeutic goals
	Disease-specific, targeted population, or general
	Available to patient and/or family members
Psychiatric medication evaluation	Psychiatric diagnosis
	Psychotropic medication recommendations
	Ongoing psychotropic medication management
	Pain management support

well accepted. Yet despite consensus statements reiterating the importance of psychosocial support in the oncology population, sufficient numbers of oncology-trained mental health professionals are not available, and heath care systems remain underresourced in this area.

PRACTITIONER BURNOUT

Working with seriously ill patients takes a substantial toll on providers from all disciplines. More than 40% of oncologists surveyed in 2012 through 2014 reported high levels of burnout (Shanafelt et al., 2014). Cancer care requires an advanced skill at managing one's own emotions, tolerating work overload, and coping with acute distress of patients and their loved ones. Feeling overwhelmed, fatigued, stressed, and depressed, and experiencing loss of enthusiasm for one's life work are all possible signs of burnout. Mental health professionals are also at risk for compassion fatigue and secondary traumatic stress reactions. Although burnout is related to the work environment, *compassion fatigue* refers to the emotional impact of caring for people who are suffering. Both are important constructs that can negatively impact patient care.

Burnout and compassion fatigue can be prevented or combatted when the work environment is structured with reasonable caseloads, sufficient time off, a practitioner culture that promotes physical and mental health, and excellent interdisciplinary coordination of care. Rarely do practitioners report that this constellation of optimal situational variables exists in the workplace. Qualitative studies indicate that it is not necessarily the sadness and emotional toll of working with patients who are acutely ill with cancer (compassion fatigue) that are cited as reasons for job dissatisfaction in oncology providers as much as an unsupportive work environment and insufficient balance between patient care and other responsibilities (burnout). It is not uncommon that mental health professionals in training aspire to work in oncology with little experience of clinical practice in the field.

As a supervisor of psychologists completing training rotation in oncology, I have found that many trainees express great enthusiasm about their wish to work with patients at the end of life, but few have had any experience in this type of work. There is often a wide disparity between the reality of providing support to families and patients with end-stage disease and how they imagined the work. Trainees express the realization that cancer can be unpredictable; they are dismayed when patients get too sick to engage in therapy die sooner than expected, and trainees feel frustrated that many people do not overtly acknowledge imminence of death. Conversely, mental health trainees often start with similar perceptions to the general population—that is, that a cancer diagnosis equals death—and they are pleasantly surprised to find that many of their patients have excellent prognoses. One of the more difficult juggling acts of psychosocial oncology involves determining how to balance the needs of new patients who seek services against established patients' need for continuity of care. A challenge in delivering mental health services lies in determining the scope of treatment. Psychological providers aim to provide care aimed at the circumscribed difficulties surrounding adjustment to the cancer diagnosis, coping with cancer, and/or addressing health-risk behaviors. People seeking mental health treatment may initially focus on topics related to their cancer care, but the potential scope is quite broad if the patient has a history of severe untreated mental health problems, substance abuse, homelessness, marital or family distress, relational issues on the job, or any of the gamut of problems that cause people to seek behavioral health treatment. The context of coping with a life-threatening diagnosis facilitates attachment and motivation to change. When patients form a strong bond with the therapist, it is difficult to switch to another provider to address broader issues that could improve their quality of life. Thus, it is important to discuss the parameters of treatment in the initial session. If the scope and model of treatment are not clear, the provider will become overwhelmed with patients who have extraordinary needs.

COUNTERTRANSFERENCE

Work with patients who have cancer is profoundly gratifying and often causes the practitioner to feel more cognizant of the finiteness of life and to be grateful for good health. At the same time, becoming attached to patients who are coping with suffering and loss takes a toll. People with personality disorders are a challenge in the context of oncology treatment because the stakes are often so high. The patient who simultaneously needs but rejects lifesaving treatment because of long-standing character logical issues is particularly vexing. Sometimes the mental health provider can be most helpful by offering perspective on how medical colleagues can communicate and work with patients who have cancer and comorbid personality disorder. Therapists may unconsciously or consciously distance themselves from suffering oncology patients. Ongoing attention to the therapist's own self-care is critical. It is difficult to predict when the therapist's caseload might coincidentally have many patients who are imminently dying. It can be particularly stressful to work with patients are similar to the therapist in age, sex, or other life circumstances.

Therapists may be tempted to disclose their personal experience with cancer or that of a family member as a way to convey empathy, but studies of self-disclosure in the medical setting indicate that it is often not helpful (Morse, McDaniel, Candib, & Beach, 2008). Conveying understanding without shifting the focus onto the provider is possible by indicating accessibility and availability (e.g., "Please call me when needed"), exploring the patient's reactions (e.g., "What was that like for you?"), and making statements (e.g., "It can be really difficult to have a parent with cancer") that indicate knowledge and empathy without personal self-disclosure. Sometimes self-disclosure is unavoidable, for example, feeling tearful if the patient is conveying particularly sad information. In instances where the therapist is able to manage their own feelings even though they are emotionally affected by the patient, self-disclosure can be helpful if the patient feels they have made an impact, felt understood, or know that the therapist cares about their well-being. Therapists undergoing their own cancer treatment or that of a close family member should carefully consider their capacity to be effective in their therapeutic role and identify whether there are any potential alternatives, such as taking time off, reducing caseload, or shifting to administrative responsibilities.

TRAINING

The field of psychosocial oncology has more clinical practitioners than any other subspecialty of health psychology. Nonetheless, it remains difficult for patients to find therapists with expertise and training in working with people diagnosed with cancer, particularly in community-based settings. From an economic perspective, creating the workforce in psychosocial oncology to meet the burgeoning population of cancer survivors and older adults with new cancer diagnoses is a pressing need. Mental health practitioners new to oncology should reach out to established organizations, such as the American Psychosocial Oncology Society, to identify potential training opportunities and mentors.

INNOVATIONS IN CLINICAL PRACTICE

The electronic medical record provides great potential for integrated, multidisciplinary cancer treatment. Mental health clinicians who document in the same electronic medical record viewed by other medical professionals can provide immense help in understanding the unique psychosocial circumstances that may affect an individual's treatment. Patients complain when they are asked the same questions repetitively and accurately report that their care is fragmented when practitioners do not communicate effectively. The electronic medical record is also fraught with peril for behavioral health specialists because a mental health diagnosis is still stigmatizing, and there is potential for loss of privacy. The permanent electronic record can be accessed by a wide range of health care providers and staff, many of whom may not have the ability to put mental health information in context. But overall, an integrated electronic medical record allows mental health clinicians to access more data to better understand the patient's history and guide treatment.

Delivery of mental health care via video conferencing or other telehealth methods is still in its earliest stages of development. This treatment modality offers many advantages, including the ability to provide evidence-based, standardized, best practice mental health assessment and treatments delivered by high-level professionals from a centralized location. The reduction in variability of mental health treatment is important because of the wide heterogeneity in the experience level of practitioners in the field. Psychiatric consultation is an example that lends itself particularly well to telemedicine because of the dearth of qualified prescribers of psychotropic medicine for this patient population.

Consider the following hypothetical example: A distressed patient needs a psychiatric evaluation quickly. The psychiatrist with specific experience in working with oncology patients conducts a video-conference assessment in conjunction with an onsite physician prescriber and onsite mental health professional trained in telemedicine. The psychiatrist consultant provides guidance to the prescriber, working from an established framework of best practice. The onsite mental health professional delivers nonpharmacologic treatment. Together, the onsite prescriber and mental health professional monitor response to psychiatric treatment and follow up at preset intervals with the specialist consultant.

Many psychiatric crises would be potentially avoidable if distressed patients were quickly assessed and appropriately treated in such a way. Many patients and practitioners have the reflexive response that telemedicine is undesirable or inferior because it seems impersonal. Yet early evidence suggests that patients in rural settings report high levels of satisfaction as well as gratitude that they do not have to travel great distance to receive high-quality care (Allen & Hayes, 2009). Some countries, such as Canada, have invested heavily in telemedicine technology. Advocates of telemedicine note that the primary barrier to effective treatment is inadequate technology, such as poor sound quality. However, sites with very-high-quality technology and experienced practitioners are able to deliver excellent telemedicine services that would be otherwise inaccessible in the community.

CONCLUSION

Progress and innovation in cancer treatment has led to increasing numbers of people living with cancer as a chronic condition. But long-term survival presents a host of psychological and behavioral challenges. Mental health professionals are needed to create holistic, integrated interventions designed to improve quality of life. Much is still to be learned about psychological approaches to prevention, screening, and early detection. Psychosocial oncology is arguably the area of medicine where clinical health psychology began and has made the greatest impact. However, similar to our medical brethren, specialty practice easily becomes insulated from other relevant cross-disciplinary work in clinical health psychology. A vast literature on psychological treatment for other acute and chronic health conditions (e.g., cardiovascular disease) that can inform psychosocial oncology remains untapped and underutilized. The foundation created by pioneers in the field of psychosocial oncology needs to be built upon, and creative psychological approaches aimed at improving outcomes in this rapidly growing patient population need to be tested. Although psychological distress is widely recognized as an impediment to effective coping, the number of available practitioners is insufficient for the demonstrated need. Appropriately trained therapists with the motivation, self-awareness, and empathy to work with people coping with cancer are needed to join the workforce to meet the needs of this rapidly growing patient population.

References

Allen, A., & Hayes, J. (2009). Patient satisfaction with teleoncology: A pilot study. *Telemedicine Journal, 1*, 41–46. http://dx.doi.org/10.1089/tmj.1.1995.1.41

American Cancer Society. (2013). *Breast cancer facts and figures 2013–2014*. Atlanta, GA: Author.

American Cancer Society. (2016). *Cancer facts and figures 2016*. Atlanta, GA: Author.

American Psychiatric Association. (2013). *Diagnostic and statistical manual of mental disorders* (5th ed.). Washington, DC: Author.

Andersen, B. L., DeRubeis, R. J., Berman, B. S., Gruman, J., Champion, V. L., Massie, M. J., . . . Rowland, J. H. (2014). Screening, assessment, and care of anxiety and depressive symptoms in adults with cancer: An American Society of Clinical Oncology guideline adaptation. *Journal of Clinical Oncology, 32*, 1605–1619. http://dx.doi.org/10.1200/JCO.2013.52.4611

Andersen, B. L., Yang, H.-C., Farrar, W. B., Golden-Kreutz, D. M., Emery, C. F., Thornton, L. M., . . . Carson, W. E., III. (2008). Psychologic intervention improves survival for breast cancer patients: A randomized clinical trial. *Cancer, 113*, 3450–3458. http://dx.doi.org/10.1002/cncr.23969

Anguiano, L., Mayer, D. K., Piven, M. L., & Rosenstein, D. (2012). A literature review of suicide in cancer patients. *Cancer Nursing, 35*, E14–E26. http://dx.doi.org/10.1097/NCC.0b013e31822fc76c

Antoni, M. H., Lehman, J. M., Kilbourn, K. M., Boyers, A. E., Culver, J. L., Alferi, S. M., . . . Carver, C. S. (2001). Cognitive-behavioral stress management intervention decreases the prevalence of depression and enhances benefit finding among women under treatment for early-stage breast cancer. *Health Psychology, 20*, 20–32. http://dx.doi.org/10.1037//0278-6133.20.1.20

Aurora, R. N., Zak, R. S., Auerbach, S. H., Casey, K. R., Chowdhuri, S., Karippot, A., . . . Morgenthaler, T. I. (2010). Best practice guide for the treatment of nightmare disorder in adults. *Journal of Clinical Sleep Medicine, 6,* 389–401.

Badr, H., Gupta, V., Sikora, A., & Posner, M. (2014). Psychological distress in patients and caregivers over the course of radiotherapy for head and neck cancer. *Oral Oncology, 50,* 1005–1011. http://dx.doi.org/10.1016/j.oraloncology.2014.07.003

Baider, L., & Surbone, A. (2010). Cancer and the family: The silent words of truth. *Journal of Clinical Oncology, 28,* 1269–1272. http://dx.doi.org/10.1200/JCO.2009.25.1223

Barrera, I., & Spiegel, D. (2014). Review of psychotherapeutic interventions on depression in cancer patients and their impact on disease progression. *International Review of Psychiatry, 26,* 31–43. http://dx.doi.org/10.3109/09540261.2013.864259

Barsevick, A. M., Dudley, W., Beck, S., Sweeney, C., Whitmer, K., & Nail, L. (2004). A randomized clinical trial of energy conservation for patients with cancer-related fatigue. *Cancer, 100,* 1302–1310. http://dx.doi.org/10.1002/cncr.20111

Beck, A. T. (1976). *Cognitive therapy and the emotional disorders.* New York, NY: International Universities Press.

Bower, J. E., Bak, K., Berger, A., Breitbart, W., Escalante, C. P., Ganz, P. A., . . . Jacobsen, P. B. (2014). Screening, assessment, and management of fatigue in adult survivors of cancer: An American Society of Clinical Oncology clinical practice guideline adaptation. *Journal of Clinical Oncology, 32,* 1840–1850. http://dx.doi.org/10.1200/JCO.2013.53.4495

Boyd, C. A., Benarroch-Gampel, J., Sheffield, K. M., Han, Y., Kuo, Y. F., & Riall, T. S. (2012). The effect of depression on stage at diagnosis, treatment, and survival in pancreatic adenocarcinoma. *Surgery, 152,* 403–413. http://dx.doi.org/10.1016/j.surg.2012.06.010

Breitbart, W., Rosenfeld, B., Gibson, C., Pessin, H., Poppito, S., Nelson, C., . . . Olden, M. (2010). Meaning-centered group psychotherapy for patients with advanced cancer: A pilot randomized controlled trial. *Psycho-Oncology, 19,* 21–28. http://dx.doi.org/10.1002/pon.1556

Breitbart, W., Rosenfeld, B., Pessin, H., Applebaum, A., Kulikowski, J., & Lichtenthal, W. G. (2015). Meaning-centered group psychotherapy: An effective intervention for improving psychological well-being in patients with advanced cancer. *Journal of Clinical Oncology, 33,* 749–754. http://dx.doi.org/10.1200/JCO.2014.57.2198

Cantarero-Villanueva, I., Fernández-Lao, C., Del Moral-Avila, R., Fernández-de-Las-Peñas, C., Feriche-Fernández-Castanys, M. B., & Arroyo-Morales, M. (2012). Effectiveness of core stability exercises and recovery myofascial release massage on fatigue in breast cancer survivors: A randomized controlled clinical trial. *Evidence-Based Complementary and Alternative Medicine, 2012,* 620619. Advance online publication. http://dx.doi.org/10.1155/2012/620619

Carlson, L. E., & Bultz, B. D. (2003). Benefits of psychosocial oncology care: Improved quality of life and medical cost offset. *Health and Quality of Life Outcomes, 1,* 8. http://dx.doi.org/10.1186/1477-7525-1-8

Chapman, B. P., Fiscella, K., Kawachi, I., Duberstein, P., & Muennig, P. (2013). Emotion suppression and mortality risk over a 12-year follow-up. *Journal of Psychosomatic Research, 75,* 381–385. http://dx.doi.org/10.1016/j.jpsychores.2013.07.014

Chen, R. C., Falchook, A. D., Tian, F., Basak, R., Hanson, L., Selvam, N., & Dusetzina, S. (2016). Aggressive care at the end-of-life for younger patients with cancer: Impact of ASCO's Choosing Wisely campaign. *Journal of Clinical Oncology, 34.* Abstract retrieved from http://ascopubs.org/doi/abs/10.1200/JCO.2016.34.18_suppl.LBA10033

Chiu, H.-Y., Huang, H.-C., Chen, P.-Y., Hou, W.-H., & Tsai, P.-S. (2015). Walking improves sleep in individuals with cancer: A meta-analysis of randomized, controlled trials. *Oncology Nursing Forum, 42,* E54–E62. http://dx.doi.org/10.1188/15.ONF.E54-E62

Chochinov, H. M. (2006). Dying, dignity, and new horizons in palliative end-of-life care. *CA: A Cancer Journal for Clinicians, 56,* 84–103. http://dx.doi.org/10.3322/canjclin.56.2.84

Clark, M. M., Atherton, P. J., Lapid, M. I., Rausch, S. M., Frost, M. H., Cheville, A. L., . . . Rummans, T. A. (2014). Caregivers of patients with cancer fatigue: A high level of symptom burden. *American Journal of Hospice and Palliative Medicine, 31,* 121–125. http://dx.doi.org/10.1177/1049909113479153

Classen, C. C., Kraemer, H. C., Blasey, C., Giese-Davis, J., Koopman, C., Palesh, O. G., . . . Spiegel, D. (2008). Supportive–expressive group therapy for primary breast cancer patients: A randomized prospective multicenter trial. *Psycho-Oncology, 17,* 438–447. http://dx.doi.org/10.1002/pon.1280

Cohen, A. B., Pierce, J. D., Jr., Chambers, J., Meade, R., Gorvine, B. J., & Koenig, H. G. (2005). Intrinsic and extrinsic religiosity, belief in the afterlife, death anxiety, and life satisfaction in young Catholics and Protestants. *Journal of Research in Personality, 39,* 307–324. http://dx.doi.org/10.1016/j.jrp.2004.02.005

Cohen, M. (2013). Cancer fatalism: Attitudes toward screening and care. In I. B. Carr & J. Steel (Eds.), *Psychological aspects of cancer* (pp. 83–99). http://dx.doi.org/10.1007/978-1-4614-4866-2_6

Cordova, M. J., Cunningham, L. C., Carlson, C. R., & Andrykowski, M. A. (2001). Posttraumatic growth following breast cancer: A controlled comparison study. *Health Psychology, 20,* 176–185.

Costanzo, E. S., Sood, A. K., & Lutgendorf, S. K. (2011). Biobehavioral influences on cancer progression. *Immunology and Allergy Clinics of North America, 31,* 109–132. http://dx.doi.org/10.1016/j.iac.2010.09.001

Craft, L. L., Vaniterson, E. H., Helenowski, I. B., Rademaker, A. W., & Courneya, K. S. (2012). Exercise effects on depressive symptoms in cancer survivors: A systematic review and meta-analysis. *Cancer Epidemiology, Biomarkers & Prevention, 21*, 3–19. http://dx.doi.org/10.1158/1055-9965.EPI-11-0634

Cramer, H., Lauche, R., Paul, A., & Dobos, G. (2012). Mindfulness-based stress reduction for breast cancer—A systematic review and meta-analysis. *Current Oncology, 19*, 343–352. http://dx.doi.org/10.3747/co.19.1016

Crist, J. V., & Grunfeld, E. A. (2013). Factors reported to influence fear of recurrence in cancer patients: A systematic review. *Psycho-Oncology, 22*, 978–986. http://dx.doi.org/10.1002/pon.3114

Dalton, S. O., Mellemkjaer, L., Olsen, J. H., Mortensen, P. B., & Johansen, C. (2002). Depression and cancer risk: A register-based study of patients hospitalized with affective disorders, Denmark, 1969–1993. *American Journal of Epidemiology, 155*, 1088–1095. http://dx.doi.org/10.1093/aje/155.12.1088

de Camargos, M. G., Paiva, C. E., Barroso, E. M., Carneseca, E. C., & Paiva, B. S. R. (2015). Understanding the differences between oncology patients and oncology health professionals concerning spirituality/religiosity: A cross-sectional study. *Medicine, 94*, e2145. http://dx.doi.org/10.1097/MD.0000000000002145

Depaola, S. J., Griffin, M., Young, J. R., & Neimeyer, R. A. (2003). Death anxiety and attitudes toward the elderly among older adults: The role of gender and ethnicity. *Death Studies, 27*, 335–354.

Dornelas, E. A., Fischer, E. H., & DiLorenzo, T. (2014). Attitudes of Black, White, and Hispanic community residents toward seeking medical help. *Race and Social Problems, 6*, 135–142. http://dx.doi.org/10.1007/s12552-014-9120-7

ECRI Institute. (2002). *ECRI evidence report: Patients' reasons for participation in clinical trials and effect of trial participation on patient outcomes.* Retrieved from https://www.ecri.org/Pages/default.aspx

Ewing, J. A. (1984). Detecting alcoholism: The CAGE questionnaire. *JAMA, 252*, 1905–10–7.

Ferrell, T., Temin, J. S., Temin, S., Alesi, E. R., Balboni, T. A., Basch, E. M., . . . Smith, T. J. (2016). *Patient and survivor care: Integration of palliative care into standard oncology care.* Retrieved from American Society of Clinical Oncology website: http://www.asco.org/practice-guidelines/quality-guidelines/guidelines/patient-and-survivor-care#/9671

Fineberg, H. V. (2008). Cancer care for the whole patient. *The Medscape Journal of Medicine, 10*, 213.

Fischer, E. H., Dornelas, E. A., & DiLorenzo, T. A. (2013). Attitudes toward seeking medical care: Development and standardization of a comprehensive scale. *Journal of Applied Social Psychology, 43*, 115–123. http://dx.doi.org/10.1111/jasp.12043

Fowler, G. (2016, June 23). Ready or not. *Genome.* Retrieved from http://genomemag.com/ready-or-not/#.WUGb_TcpBhE

Friedenreich, C. M., Neilson, H. K., Farris, M. S., & Courneya, K. C. (2016). Physical activity and cancer outcomes: A precision medicine approach. *Clinical Cancer Research.* http://dx.doi.org/10.1158/1078-0432.CCR-16-0067

Ganz, P. A. (2016). Understanding the impact of breast cancer adjuvant endocrine therapy on cognitive function: A work in progress. *British Journal of Cancer, 114,* 953–955. http://dx.doi.org/10.1038/bjc.2016.89

Garland, S. N., Johnson, J. A., Savard, J., Gehrman, P., Perlis, M., Carlson, L., & Campbell, T. (2014). Sleeping well with cancer: A systematic review of cognitive behavioral therapy for insomnia in cancer patients. *Neuropsychiatric Disease and Treatment, 10,* 1113–1124.

Geirdal, A. O., & Dahl, A. A. (2008). The relationship between coping strategies and anxiety in women from families with familial breast–ovarian cancer in the absence of demonstrated mutations. *Psycho-Oncology, 17,* 49–57. http://dx.doi.org/10.1002/pon.1198

Girgis, A., Lambert, S. D., McElduff, P., Bonevski, B., Lecathelinais, C., Boyes, A., & Stacey, F. (2013). Some things change, some things stay the same: A longitudinal analysis of cancer caregivers' unmet supportive care needs. *Psycho-Oncology, 22,* 1557–1564. http://dx.doi.org/10.1002/pon.3166

Gray, P. J., Lin, C. C., Jemal, A., & Efstathiou, J. (2014). Recent trends in the management of localized prostate cancer: Results from the National Cancer Data Base. *Journal of Clinical Oncology, 32,* Abstract 5066. Retrieved from American Society of Clinical Oncology website: http://meetinglibrary.asco.org/content/130897-144

Greenberg, D. B. (2011). The signal of suicide rates seen from a distance in patients with pancreatic cancer. *Cancer, 117,* 446–448. http://dx.doi.org/10.1002/cncr.25419

Greenlee, H., Balneaves, L. G., Carlson, L. E., Cohen, M., Deng, G., Hershman, D., . . . Tripathy, D. (2014). Clinical practice guidelines on the use of integrative therapies as supportive care in patients treated for breast cancer. *Journal of the National Cancer Institute Monographs, 2014,* 346–358. http://dx.doi.org/10.1093/jncimonographs/lgu041

Greenstein, M. (2000). The house that's on fire: Meaning-centered psychotherapy pilot group for cancer patients. *American Journal of Psychotherapy, 54,* 501–511.

Greer, J. A., Graham, J. S., & Safren, S. A. (2010). Resolving treatment complications associated with comorbid medical conditions. In M. W. Otto & S. G. Hofmann (Eds.), *Avoiding treatment failures in the anxiety disorders* (pp. 317–346). New York, NY: Springer.

Greer, J. A., Park, E. R., Prigerson, H. G., & Safren, S. A. (2010). Tailoring cognitive-behavioral therapy to treat anxiety comorbid with advanced cancer. *Journal of Cognitive Psychotherapy*, *24*, 294–313. http://dx.doi.org/10.1891/0889-8391.24.4.294

Grossi, E., Groth, N., Mosconi, P., Cerutti, R., Pace, F., Compare, A., & Apolone, G. (2006). Development and validation of the short version of the Psychological General Well-Being Index (PGWB-S). *Health and Quality of Life Outcomes*, *4*, 88. http://dx.doi.org/10.1186/1477-7525-4-88

Guy, G. P., Jr., Berkowitz, Z., Tai, E., Holman, D. M., Everett Jones, S., & Richardson, L. (2014). Indoor tanning among high school students in the United States, 2009 and 2011. *JAMA Dermatology*, *150*, 501–511.

Haley, W. E., Roth, D. L., Howard, G., & Safford, M. M. (2010). Caregiving strain and estimated risk for stroke and coronary heart disease among spouse caregivers: Differential effects by race and sex. *Stroke*, *41*, 331–336. http://dx.doi.org/10.1161/STROKEAHA.109.568279

Hart, S. L., Hoyt, M. A., Diefenbach, M., Anderson, D. R., Kilbourn, K. M., Craft, L. L., . . . Stanton, A. L. (2012). Meta-analysis of efficacy of interventions for elevated depressive symptoms in adults diagnosed with cancer. *Journal of the National Cancer Institute*, *104*, 990–1004. http://dx.doi.org/10.1093/jnci/djs256

He, W., Goodkind, D., & Kowal, P. (2016). An aging world: 2015 International Population Reports. *International Population Reports*. Washington, DC: U.S. Government Publishing Office.

Heston, A.-H., Schwartz, A. L., Justice-Gardiner, H., & Hohman, K. H. (2015). Addressing physical activity needs of survivors by developing a community-based exercise program: LIVESTRONG® at the YMCA. *Clinical Journal of Oncology Nursing*, *19*, 213–217. http://dx.doi.org/10.1188/15.CJON.213-217

Hinton, J. (1994). Can home care maintain an acceptable quality of life for patients with terminal cancer and their relatives? *Palliative Medicine*, *8*, 183–196. http://dx.doi.org/10.1177/026921639400800302

Hirsch, J. K., Molnar, D., Chang, E. C., & Sirois, F. M. (2015). Future orientation and health quality of life in primary care: Vitality as a mediator. *Quality of Life Research*, *24*, 1653–1659. http://dx.doi.org/10.1007/s11136-014-0901-7

Hodges, K., & Winstanley, S. (2012). Effects of optimism, social support, fighting spirit, cancer worry and internal health locus of control on positive affect in cancer survivors: A path analysis. *Stress and Health*, *28*, 408–415. http://dx.doi.org/10.1002/smi.2471

Holland, J. C., Greenberg, D. C., & Hughes, M. K. (2006). *Quick reference guide for oncology clinicians: The psychiatric and psychological dimensions of cancer symptom management*. Charlottesville, VA: American Psychosocial Oncology Society.

Hopko, D. R., Robertson, S. M. C., & Colman, L. (2008). Behavioral activation therapy for depressed cancer patients: Factors associated with treatment outcome and attrition. *International Journal of Behavioral Consultation and Therapy, 4,* 319–327. http://dx.doi.org/10.1037/h0100862

International Human Genome Sequencing Consortium. (2004). Finishing the euchromatic sequence of the human genome. *Nature, 431,* 931–945. http://dx.doi.org/10.1038/nature03001

Jacobson, N. S., Martell, C. R., & Dimidjian, S. (2001). Behavioral activation treatment for depression: Returning to contextual roots. *Clinical Psychology: Science and Practice, 8,* 255–270. http://dx.doi.org/10.1093/clipsy.8.3.255

Jones, J. M. (2013). *In U.S., 40% get less than recommended amount of sleep.* Retrieved from http://www.gallup.com/poll/166553/less-recommended-amount-sleep. aspx

Kane, L. (2014). *Medscape ethics report 2014, Part 1: Life, death and pain.* Retrieved from http://www.medscape.com/features/slideshow/public/ethics2014-part2

Kaplow, R. (2005). Sleep deprivation and psychosocial impact in acutely ill cancer patients. *Critical Care Nursing Clinics of North America, 17,* 225–237. http://dx.doi.org/10.1016/j.ccell.2005.04.010

Karr, K. (2008). *Crazy, sexy cancer survivor.* Charleston, SC: Skirt!

Kavalieratos, D., Corbelli, J., Zhang, D., Dionne-Odom, J. N., Ernecoff, N. C., Hanmer, J., . . . Schenker, Y. (2016). Association between palliative care and patient and caregiver outcomes: A systematic review and meta-analysis. *JAMA, 316,* 2104–2114.

Kim, S. W. (2011). Prostatic disease and sexual dysfunction. *Korean Journal of Urology, 52,* 373–378. http://dx.doi.org/10.4111/kju.2011.52.6.373

Kissane, D. W., Grabsch, B., Clarke, D. M., Smith, G. C., Love, A. W., Bloch, S., . . . Li, Y. (2007). Supportive–expressive group therapy for women with metastatic breast cancer: Survival and psychosocial outcome from a randomized controlled trial. *Psycho-Oncology, 16,* 277–286. http://dx.doi.org/10.1002/pon.1185

Klonsky, E. D., & May, A. M. (2015, August 31). Impulsivity and suicide risk: Review and clinical implications. Retrieved from http://www.cancernetwork. com/special-reports/impulsivity-and-suicide-risk-review-and-clinical-implications/page/0/3

Koontz, B. F., Flynn, K., Reese, J. B., Urdeneta, A. I., Moghanaki, D., & Porter, L. S. (2012). Significant variation in provider discussion of sexual side effects with radiation therapy patients. *International Journal of Radiation Oncology Biology Physics, 84,* 2–3.

Kotsopoulos, J., Chen, W. Y., Gates, M. A., Tworoger, S. S., Hankinson, S. E., & Rosner, B. A. (2010). Risk factors for ductal and lobular breast cancer: Results from the Nurses' Health Study. *Breast Cancer Research, 12,* R106.

Krebber, A. M. H., Buffart, L. M., Kleijn, G., Riepma, I. C., de Bree, R., Leemans, C. R., . . . Verdonck-de Leeuw, I. M. (2014). Prevalence of depression in cancer patients: A meta-analysis of diagnostic interviews and self-report instruments. *Psycho-Oncology, 23,* 121–130. http://dx.doi.org/10.1002/pon.3409

Kroenke, K., & Spitzer, R. L. (2002). The PHQ-9: A new depression diagnostic and severity measure. *Psychiatric Annals, 32,* 509–515. http://dx.doi.org/10.3928/0048-5713-20020901-06

Kummerow, K. L., Du, L., Penson, D. F., Shyr, Y., & Hooks, M. A. (2015). Nationwide trends in mastectomy for early-stage breast cancer. *JAMA Surgery, 150,* 9–16. http://dx.doi.org/10.1001/jamasurg.2014.2895

Kushi, L. H., Doyle, C., McCullough, M., Rock, C. L., Demark-Wahnefried, W., Bandera, E. V., . . . Gansler, T. (2012). American Cancer Society guidelines on nutrition and physical activity for cancer prevention: Reducing the risk of cancer with healthy food choices and physical activity. *CA: A Cancer Journal for Clinicians, 62,* 30–67. http://dx.doi.org/10.3322/caac.20140

Lancaster, T., & Stead, L. F. (2017). Individual behavioural counselling for smoking cessation. *Cochrane Database of Systematic Reviews, 2017*(3). http://dx.doi.org/10.1002/14651858.CD001292.pub3

Latini, D. M., Hart, S. L., Knight, S. J., Cowan, J. E., Ross, P. L., Duchane, J., . . . The CaPSURE Investigators. (2007). The relationship between anxiety and time to treatment for patients with prostate cancer on surveillance. *The Journal of Urology, 178,* 823–831. http://dx.doi.org/10.1016/j.juro.2007.05.039

Lebel, S., Maheu, C., Lefebvre, M., Secord, S., Courbasson, C., Singh, M., . . . Catton, P. (2014). Addressing fear of cancer recurrence among women with cancer: A feasibility and preliminary outcome study. *Journal of Cancer Survivorship: Research and Practice, 8,* 485–496. http://dx.doi.org/10.1007/s11764-014-0357-3

Lehto, U. S., Ojanen, M., Dyba, T., Aromaa, A., & Kellokumpu-Lehtinen, P. (2007). Baseline psychosocial predictors of survival in localized melanoma. *Journal of Psychosomatic Research, 63,* 9–15. http://dx.doi.org/10.1016/j.jpsychores.2007.01.001

Lejuez, C. W., Hopko, D. R., Acierno, R., Daughters, S. B., & Pagoto, S. L. (2011). Ten-year revision of the brief behavioral activation treatment for depression: Revised treatment manual. *Behavior Modification, 35,* 111–161. http://dx.doi.org/10.1177/0145445510390929

Lerman, C., Lustbader, E., Rimer, B., Daly, M., Miller, S., Sands, C., & Balshem, A. (1995). Effects of individualized breast cancer risk counseling: A randomized trial. *Journal of the National Cancer Institute, 87,* 286–292. http://dx.doi.org/10.1093/jnci/87.4.286

Linden, W., Vodermaier, A., MacKenzie, R., & Greig, D. (2012). Anxiety and depression after cancer diagnosis: Prevalence rates by cancer type, gender, and age. *Journal of Affective Disorders, 141,* 343–351. http://dx.doi.org/10.1016/j.jad.2012.03.025

Lindner, O. C., Phillips, B., McCabe, M. G., Mayes, A., Wearden, A., Varese, F., & Talmi, D. (2014). A meta-analysis of cognitive impairment following adult cancer chemotherapy. *Neuropsychology, 28,* 726–740. http://dx.doi.org/10.1037/neu0000064

Liu, Y., Pérez, M., Aft, R. L., Massman, K., Robinson, E., Myles, S., . . . Jeffe, D. B. (2010). Accuracy of perceived risk of recurrence among patients with early-stage breast cancer. *Cancer Epidemiology, Biomarkers & Prevention, 19,* 675–680. http://dx.doi.org/10.1158/1055-9965.EPI-09-1051

Loren, A. W., Mangu, P. B., Beck, L. N., Brennan, L., Magdalinski, A. J., Partridge, A. H., . . . Wallace, W. H. (2013). Fertility preservation for patients with cancer: American Society of Clinical Oncology clinical practice guideline update. *Journal of Clinical Oncology, 31,* 2500–2510. http://dx.doi.org/10.1200/JCO.2013.49.2678

Low, C. A., & Stanton, A. L. (2015). Activity disruption and depressive symptoms in women living with metastatic breast cancer. *Health Psychology, 34,* 89–92. http://dx.doi.org/10.1037/hea0000052

Lutgendorf, S. K., Sood, A. K., & Antoni, M. H. (2010). Host factors and cancer progression: Biobehavioral signaling pathways and interventions. *Journal of Clinical Oncology, 28,* 4094–4099. http://dx.doi.org/10.1200/JCO.2009.26.9357

Maiorino, M. I., Chiodini, P., Bellastella, G., Giugliano, D., & Esposito, K. (2016). Sexual dysfunction in women with cancer: A systematic review with meta-analysis of studies using the Female Sexual Function Index. *Endocrine, 54,* 329–341. http://dx.doi.org/10.1007/s12020-015-0812-6

Manne, S. L., Ostroff, J. S., Norton, T. R., Fox, K., Goldstein, L., & Grana, G. (2006). Cancer-related relationship communication in couples coping with early stage breast cancer. *Psycho-Oncology, 15,* 234–247. http://dx.doi.org/10.1002/pon.941

Manne, S. L., Ostroff, J. S., Winkel, G., Grana, G., & Fox, K. (2005). Partner unsupportive responses, avoidant coping, and distress among women with early stage breast cancer: Patient and partner perspectives. *Health Psychology, 24,* 635–641. http://dx.doi.org/10.1037/0278-6133.24.6.635

Maruvka, Y. E., Tang, M., & Michor, F. (2014). On the validity of using increases in 5-year survival rates to measure success in the fight against cancer. *PLoS One, 9,* e83100. http://dx.doi.org/10.1371/journal.pone.0083100

Marvin, N. (Producer), & Darabout, F. (Director). (1994). *The Shawshank redemption* [Motion picture]. United States: Castle Rock Entertainment.

Massie, M. J. (2004). Prevalence of depression in patients with cancer. *Journal of the National Cancer Institute Monographs, 32,* 57–71. http://dx.doi.org/10.1093/jncimonographs/lgh014

McDaniel, S. H., Doherty, W. J., & Hepworth, J. (2014). *Medical family therapy and integrated care* (2nd ed.). http://dx.doi.org/10.1037/14256-000

Mehnert, A., Brähler, E., Faller, H., Härter, M., Keller, M., Schulz, H., . . . Koch, U. (2014). Four-week prevalence of mental disorders in patients with cancer across major tumor entities. *Journal of Clinical Oncology, 32,* 3540–3546. http://dx.doi.org/10.1200/JCO.2014.56.0086

Meijer, A., Roseman, M., Milette, K., Coyne, J. C., Stefanek, M. E., Ziegelstein, R. C., . . . Thombs, B. D. (2011). Depression screening and patient outcomes in cancer: A systematic review. *PLoS One, 6,* e27181. http://dx.doi.org/10.1371/journal.pone.0027181

Meyers, F. J., Carducci, M., Loscalzo, M. J., Linder, J., Greasby, T., & Beckett, L. A. (2011). Effects of a problem-solving intervention (COPE) on quality of life for patients with advanced cancer on clinical trials and their caregivers: Simultaneous care educational intervention (SCEI): Linking palliation and clinical trials. *Journal of Palliative Medicine, 14,* 465–473. http://dx.doi.org/10.1089/jpm.2010.0416

Misono, S., Weiss, N. S., Fann, J. R., Redman, M., & Yueh, B. (2008). Incidence of suicide in persons with cancer. *Journal of Clinical Oncology, 26,* 4731–4738. http://dx.doi.org/10.1200/JCO.2007.13.8941

Mitchell, A. J. (2008). Are one or two simple questions sufficient to detect depression in cancer and palliative care? A Bayesian meta-analysis. *British Journal of Cancer, 98,* 1934–1943. http://dx.doi.org/10.1038/sj.bjc.6604396

Mitchell, A. J., Ferguson, D. W., Gill, J., Paul, J., & Symonds, P. (2013). Depression and anxiety in long-term cancer survivors compared with spouses and healthy controls: A systematic review and meta-analysis. *The Lancet Oncology, 14,* 721–732. http://dx.doi.org/10.1016/S1470-2045(13)70244-4

Morse, D. S., McDaniel, S. H., Candib, L. M., & Beach, M. C. (2008). "Enough about me, let's get back to you": Physician self-disclosure during primary care encounters. *Annals of Internal Medicine, 149,* 835–837. http://dx.doi.org/10.7326/0003-4819-149-11-200812020-00015

Mosher, C. E., & Danoff-Burg, S. (2010). Addiction to indoor tanning: Relation to anxiety, depression, and substance use. *JAMA Dermatology, 146,* 412–417.

Moyer, V. A., & U.S. Preventive Services Task Force. (2014). Screening for lung cancer: U.S. Preventive Services Task Force recommendation statement. *Annals of Internal Medicine, 160,* 330–338. http://dx.doi.org/10.7326/M13-2771

National Hospice and Palliative Care Organization. (2014). *NHPCO's facts and figures: Hospice care in America.* Retrieved from https://www.nhpco.org/sites/default/files/public/Statistics_Research/2014_Facts_Figures.pdf

National Sleep Foundation. (2015). *National Sleep Foundation recommends new sleep times* [Press release]. Retrieved from https://sleepfoundation.org/press-release/national-sleep-foundation-recommends-new-sleep-times

Ng, C. G., Boks, M. P. M., Zainal, N. Z., & de Wit, N. J. (2011). The prevalence and pharmacotherapy of depression in cancer patients. *Journal of Affective Disorders, 131*, 1–7. http://dx.doi.org/10.1016/j.jad.2010.07.034

Northouse, L. L., Katapodi, M. C., Song, L., Zhang, L., & Mood, D. W. (2010). Interventions with family caregivers of cancer patients: Meta-analysis of randomized trials. *CA: A Cancer Journal for Clinicians, 60*, 317–339.

Osborn, R. L., Demoncada, A. C., & Feuerstein, M. (2006). Psychosocial interventions for depression, anxiety, and quality of life in cancer survivors: Meta-analyses. *International Journal of Psychiatry in Medicine, 36*, 13–34. http://dx.doi.org/10.2190/EUFN-RV1K-Y3TR-FK0L

Otte, J. L., Carpenter, J. S., Manchanda, S., Rand, K. L., Skaar, T. C., Weaver, M., ... Landis, C. (2015). Systematic review of sleep disorders in cancer patients: Can the prevalence of sleep disorders be ascertained? *Cancer Medicine, 4*, 183–200. http://dx.doi.org/10.1002/cam4.356

Ozga, M., Aghajanian, C., Myers-Virtue, S., McDonnell, G., Jhanwar, S., Hichenberg, S., & Sulimanoff, I. (2015). A systematic review of ovarian cancer and fear of recurrence. *Palliative & Supportive Care, 13*, 1771–1780. http://dx.doi.org/10.1017/S1478951515000127

Partridge, A., Adloff, K., Blood, E., Dees, E. C., Kaelin, C., Golshan, M., ... Winer, E. (2008). Risk perceptions and psychosocial outcomes of women with ductal carcinoma in situ: Longitudinal results from a cohort study. *Journal of the National Cancer Institute, 100*, 243–251. http://dx.doi.org/10.1093/jnci/djn010

Penedo, F. J., Dahn, J. R., Kinsinger, D., Antoni, M. H., Molton, I., Gonzalez, J. S., ... Schneiderman, N. (2006). Anger suppression mediates the relationship between optimism and natural killer cell cytotoxicity in men treated for localized prostate cancer. *Journal of Psychosomatic Research, 60*, 423–427. http://dx.doi.org/10.1016/j.jpsychores.2005.08.001

Pinquart, M., & Duberstein, P. R. (2010). Depression and cancer mortality: A meta-analysis. *Psychological Medicine, 40*, 1797–1810. http://dx.doi.org/10.1017/S0033291709992285

Prati, G., & Pietrantoni, L. (2009). Optimism, social support, and coping strategies as factors contributing to posttraumatic growth: A meta-analysis. *Journal of Loss and Trauma, 14*, 364–388. http://dx.doi.org/10.1080/15325020902724271

Prue, G., Rankin, J., Allen, J., Gracey, J., & Cramp, F. (2006). Cancer-related fatigue: A critical appraisal. *European Journal of Cancer, 42*, 846–863. http://dx.doi.org/10.1016/j.ejca.2005.11.026

Rajotte, E. J., Yi, J. C., Baker, K. S., Gregerson, L., Leiserowitz, A., & Syrjala, K. L. (2012). Community-based exercise program effectiveness and safety for cancer survivors. *Journal of Cancer Survivorship: Research and Practice, 6,* 219–228. http://dx.doi.org/10.1007/s11764-011-0213-7

Rapaport, M. H., Schettler, P., & Bresee, C. (2012). A preliminary study of the effects of repeated massage on hypothalamic–pituitary–adrenal and immune function in healthy individuals: A study of mechanisms of action and dosage. *Journal of Alternative and Complementary Medicine, 18,* 789–797. http://dx.doi.org/10.1089/acm.2011.0071

Regan, T. W., Lambert, S. D., Girgis, A., Kelly, B., Kayser, K., & Turner, J. (2012). Do couple-based interventions make a difference for couples affected by cancer? A systematic review. *BMC Cancer, 12,* 279. http://dx.doi.org/10.1186/1471-2407-12-279

Reyna, V. F., Nelson, W. L., Han, P. K., & Dieckmann, N. F. (2009). How numeracy influences risk comprehension and medical decision making. *Psychological Bulletin, 135,* 943–973. http://dx.doi.org/10.1037/a0017327

Reyna, V. F., Nelson, W. L., Han, P. K., & Pignone, M. P. (2015). Decision making and cancer. *American Psychologist, 70,* 105–118. http://dx.doi.org/10.1037/a0036834

Reynolds, P., Hurley, S., Torres, M., Jackson, J., Boyd, P., & Chen, V. W. (2000). Use of coping strategies and breast cancer survival: Results from the Black/White Cancer Survival Study. *American Journal of Epidemiology, 152,* 940–949. http://dx.doi.org/10.1093/aje/152.10.940

Rosenfeld, B., Pessin, H., Marziliano, A., Jacobson, C., Sorger, B., Abbey, J., . . . Breitbart, W. (2014). Does desire for hastened death change in terminally ill cancer patients? *Social Science & Medicine, 111,* 35–40. http://dx.doi.org/10.1016/j.socscimed.2014.03.027

Rustøen, T., Cooper, B. A., & Miaskowski, C. (2011). A longitudinal study of the effects of a hope intervention on levels of hope and psychological distress in a community-based sample of oncology patients. *European Journal of Oncology Nursing, 15,* 351–357. http://dx.doi.org/10.1016/j.ejon.2010.09.001

Saad, L. (2013). *U.S. support for euthanasia hinges on how it's described* [2013 Gallup poll]. Retrieved from http://www.gallup.com/poll/162815/support-euthanasia-hinges-described.aspx

Sabariego, C., Brach, M., Herschbach, P., Berg, P., & Stucki, G. (2011). Cost-effectiveness of cognitive-behavioral group therapy for dysfunctional fear of progression in cancer patients. *The European Journal of Health Economics, 12,* 489–497. http://dx.doi.org/10.1007/s10198-010-0266-y

Sarkar, S., Scherwath, A., Schirmer, L., Schulz-Kindermann, F., Neumann, K., Kruse, M., . . . Mehnert, A. (2014). Fear of recurrence and its impact on quality of life in patients with hematological cancers in the course of allogeneic hematopoietic SCT. *Bone Marrow Transplantation, 49*, 1217–1222. http://dx.doi.org/10.1038/bmt.2014.139

Savard, J., Simard, S., Blanchet, J., Ivers, H., & Morin, C. M. (2001). Prevalence, clinical characteristics, and risk factors for insomnia in the context of breast cancer. *Sleep, 24*, 583–590. http://dx.doi.org/10.1093/sleep/24.5.583

Schnarch, D. (1997). *Passionate marriage: Keeping love and intimacy alive in committed relationships.* New York, NY: Norton.

Schover, L. R., Fouladi, R. T., Warneke, C. L., Neese, L., Klein, E. A., Zippe, C., & Kupelian, P. A. (2002). Defining sexual outcomes after treatment for localized prostate carcinoma. *Cancer, 95*, 1773–1785. http://dx.doi.org/10.1002/cncr.10848

ScienceDaily. (2008). *Most physicians sleep fewer hours than needed for peak performance, report says.* Retrieved from https://www.sciencedaily.com/releases/2008/03/080304075723.htm

Shanafelt, T. D., Gradishar, W. J., Kosty, M., Satele, D., Chew, H., Horn, L., . . . Raymond, M. (2014). Burnout and career satisfaction among U.S. oncologists. *Journal of Clinical Oncology, 32*, 678–686. http://dx.doi.org/10.1200/JCO.2013.51.8480

Silver, J. K., Baima, J., & Mayer, R. S. (2013). Impairment-driven cancer rehabilitation: An essential component of quality care and survivorship. *CA: A Cancer Journal for Clinicians, 63*, 295–317. http://dx.doi.org/10.3322/caac.21186

Simard, S., Thewes, B., Humphris, G., Dixon, M., Hayden, C., Mireskandari, S., & Ozakinci, G. (2013). Fear of cancer recurrence in adult cancer survivors: A systematic review of quantitative studies. *Journal of Cancer Survivorship: Research and Practice, 7*, 300–322. http://dx.doi.org/10.1007/s11764-013-0272-z

Simpson, J. S., Carlson, L. E., & Trew, M. E. (2001). Effect of group therapy for breast cancer on healthcare utilization. *Cancer Practice, 9*, 19–26. http://dx.doi.org/10.1046/j.1523-5394.2001.91005.x

Smith, T. W., Glazer, K., Ruiz, J. M., & Gallo, L. C. (2004). Hostility, anger, aggressiveness, and coronary heart disease: An interpersonal perspective on personality, emotion, and health. *Journal of Personality, 72*, 1217–1270. http://dx.doi.org/10.1111/j.1467-6494.2004.00296.x

Snyder, C. R., Rand, K. L., & Sigmon, D. R. (2002). Hope theory: A member of the positive psychology family. In C. R. Snyder & S. J. Lopez (Eds.), *Handbook of positive psychology* (pp. 257–276). New York, NY: Oxford University Press.

Song, M., & Giovannucci, E. (2016). Preventable incidence and mortality of carcinoma associated with lifestyle factors among White adults in the United States. *JAMA Oncology, 2*, 2374–2437. http://dx.doi.org/10.1001/jamaoncol.2016.0843

Spiegel, D., Kraemer, H. C., Bloom, J. R., & Gottheil, E. (1989). Effect of psycho-social treatment on survival of patients with metastatic breast cancer. *The Lancet, 334,* 888–891. http://dx.doi.org/10.1016/S0140-6736(89)91551-1

Spitzer, R. L., Kroenke, K., & Williams, J. B. (1999). Validation and utility of a self-report version of PRIME-MD: The PHQ primary care study. *JAMA, 282,* 1737–1744. http://dx.doi.org/10.1001/jama.282.18.1737

Stanton, A. L., Danoff-Burg, S., Cameron, C. L., Bishop, M., Collins, C. A., Kirk, S. B., . . . Twillman, R. (2000). Emotionally expressive coping predicts psychological and physical adjustment to breast cancer. *Journal of Consulting and Clinical Psychology, 68,* 875–882. http://dx.doi.org/10.1037/0022-006X.68.5.875

Stark, D., Kiely, M., Smith, A., Velikova, G., House, A., & Selby, P. (2002). Anxiety disorders in cancer patients: Their nature, associations, and relation to quality of life. *Journal of Clinical Oncology, 20,* 3137–3148. http://dx.doi.org/10.1200/JCO.2002.08.549

Stead, M. L., Brown, J. M., Fallowfield, L., & Selby, P. (2003). Lack of communication between healthcare professionals and women with ovarian cancer about sexual issues. *British Journal of Cancer, 88,* 666–671. http://dx.doi.org/10.1038/sj.bjc.6600799

Steel, J. L., Geller, D. A., Gamblin, T. C., Olek, M. C., & Carr, B. I. (2007). Depression, immunity, and survival in patients with hepatobiliary carcinoma. *Journal of Clinical Oncology, 25,* 2397–2405. http://dx.doi.org/10.1200/JCO.2006.06.4592

Step, M. M., Kypriotakis, G. M., & Rose, J. H. (2013). An exploration of the relative influence of patient's age and cancer recurrence status on symptom distress, anxiety, and depression over time. *Journal of Psychosocial Oncology, 31,* 168–190. http://dx.doi.org/10.1080/07347332.2012.761318

Swencionis, C., Wylie-Rosett, J., Lent, M. R., Ginsberg, M., Cimino, C., Wassertheil-Smoller, S., . . . Segal-Isaacson, C. J. (2013). Weight change, psychological well-being, and vitality in adults participating in a cognitive-behavioral weight loss program. *Health Psychology, 32,* 439–446. http://dx.doi.org/10.1037/a0029186

Thekkumpurath, P., Walker, J., Butcher, I., Hodges, L., Kleiboer, A., O'Connor, M., . . . Sharpe, M. (2011). Screening for major depression in cancer outpatients: The diagnostic accuracy of the 9-item patient health questionnaire. *Cancer, 117,* 218–227. http://dx.doi.org/10.1002/cncr.25514

Thornton, L. M., Cheavens, J. S., Heitzmann, C. A., Dorfman, C. S., Wu, S. M., & Andersen, B. L. (2014). Test of mindfulness and hope components in a psychological intervention for women with cancer recurrence. *Journal of Consulting and Clinical Psychology, 82,* 1087–1100. http://dx.doi.org/10.1037/a0036959

Traa, M. J., De Vries, J., Roukema, J. A., & Den Oudsten, B. L. (2012). Sexual (dys) function and the quality of sexual life in patients with colorectal cancer: A systematic review. *Annals of Oncology, 23,* 19–27. http://dx.doi.org/10.1093/annonc/mdr133

Tralongo, P., Annunziata, M. A., Santoro, A., Tirelli, U., & Surbone, A. (2013). Beyond semantics: The need to better categorize patients with cancer. *Journal of Clinical Oncology, 31,* 2637–2638. http://dx.doi.org/10.1200/JCO.2013.50.0850

Tripp, M. K., Watson, M., Balk, S. J., Swetter, S. M., & Gershenwald, J. E. (2016). State of the science on prevention and screening to reduce melanoma incidence and mortality: The time is now. *CA: A Cancer Journal for Clinicians, 66,* 460–480. Advance online publication. http://dx.doi.org/10.3322/caac.21352

Vanderbilt University. (2010). *How cancer cells lose their (circadian) rhythm.* Retrieved from https://www.sciencedaily.com/releases/2010/05/100510151344.htm

Vos, M. S., Putter, H., van Houwelingen, H. C., & de Haes, H. C. J. M. (2008). Denial in lung cancer patients: A longitudinal study. *Psycho-Oncology, 17,* 1163–1171. http://dx.doi.org/10.1002/pon.1325

Walker, J., Hansen, C. H., Martin, P., Symeonides, S., Ramessur, R., Murray, G., & Sharpe, M. (2014). Prevalence, associations, and adequacy of treatment of major depression in patients with cancer: A cross-sectional analysis of routinely collected clinical data. *The Lancet: Psychiatry, 1,* 343–350. http://dx.doi.org/10.1016/S2215-0366(14)70313-X

Walker, J., Waters, R. A., Murray, G., Swanson, H., Hibberd, C. J., Rush, R. W., . . . Sharpe, M. (2008). Better off dead: Suicidal thoughts in cancer patients. *Journal of Clinical Oncology, 26,* 4725–4730. http://dx.doi.org/10.1200/JCO.2007.11.8844

Wassertheil-Smoller, S., Arredondo, E. M., Cai, J., Castaneda, S. F., Choca, J. P., Gallo, L. C., . . . Zee, P. C. (2014). Depression, anxiety, antidepressant use, and cardiovascular disease among Hispanic men and women of different national backgrounds: Results from the Hispanic Community Health Study/Study of Latinos. *Annals of Epidemiology, 24,* 822–830. http://dx.doi.org/10.1016/j.annepidem.2014.09.003

Watkins, E. R., Mullan, E., Wingrove, J., Rimes, K., Steiner, H., Bathurst, N., . . . Scott, J. (2011). Rumination-focused cognitive-behavioural therapy for residual depression: Phase II randomised controlled trial. *The British Journal of Psychiatry, 199,* 317–322. http://dx.doi.org/10.1192/bjp.bp.110.090282

Weis, R., & Speridakos, E. C. (2011). A meta-analysis of hope enhancement strategies in clinical and community settings. *Psychology of Well-Being: Theory, Research and Practice, 5,* 1–16.

Welch, H. G., & Robertson, D. J. (2016). Colorectal cancer on the decline—Why screening can't explain it all. *The New England Journal of Medicine, 374,* 1605–1607. http://dx.doi.org/10.1056/NEJMp1600448

Welch, H. G., Schwartz, L., & Woloshin, S. (2011). *Over-diagnosed: Making people sick in the pursuit of health.* Boston, MA: Beacon Press Books.

Wellisch, D. K., & Cohen, M. (2011). In the midnight hour: Cancer and nightmares. A review of theories and interventions in psycho-oncology. *Palliative & Supportive Care, 9,* 191–200. http://dx.doi.org/10.1017/S147895151100006X

Wiechno, P., Demkow, T., Kubiak, K., Sadowska, M., & Kaminska, J. (2007). The quality of life and hormonal disturbances in testicular cancer survivors in Cisplatin era. *European Urology, 52,* 1448–1455. http://dx.doi.org/10.1016/j.eururo.2007.05.012

Wu, Y. P., Aspinwall, L. G., Conn, B. M., Stump, T., Grahmann, B., & Leachman, S. A. (2016). A systematic review of interventions to improve adherence to melanoma preventive behaviors for individuals at elevated risk. *Preventive Medicine, 88,* 153–167. http://dx.doi.org/10.1016/j.ypmed.2016.04.010

Yeung, A., & Kam, R. (2006). *Recognizing and treating depression in Asian Americans.* Retrieved from http://www.psychiatrictimes.com/display/article/10168/51621

Zhang, A. Y., Gary, F., & Zhu, H. (2015). Exploration of depressive symptoms in African American cancer patients. *Journal of Mental Health, 24,* 351–356. http://dx.doi.org/10.3109/09638237.2014.998806

Index

About the Author

Ellen A. Dornelas, PhD, is the director for cancer clinical research at Hartford Healthcare Cancer Institute in Connecticut and associate professor of clinical medicine at the University of Connecticut School of Medicine. Dr. Dornelas received her degree in health psychology from Ferkauf Graduate School of Psychology, Yeshiva University, New York, NY. She has focused her career on the integration of practice and research in clinical health psychology. Dr. Dornelas is recognized for her expertise in treating people with heart disease as well as cancer. She has supervised and mentored students for over two decades. Dr. Dornelas has authored multiple books and journal articles and is a featured guest expert on APA's Psychotherapy Video Series. She is a Fellow in the American Psychological Association's Division 29 (Society for the Advancement of Psychotherapy) and a practicing psychotherapist.